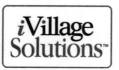

6 *weeks to*
LOSING IT FOR GOOD

Edited by Emily Lapkin

with Liz Neporent, M.A., and Lynn Grieger, R.D., C.D.E.

RUTLEDGE HILL PRESS™

Nashville, Tennessee

A Division of Thomas Nelson, Inc.

www.ThomasNelson.com

The information in this book is for general knowledge only. Before beginning this or any other diet and exercise program, consult with your personal physician. Seek prompt medical care for any specific medical problem or concern.

Published by Rutledge Hill Press, a Division of Thomas Nelson, Inc., P.O. Box 141000, Nashville, Tennessee 37214.

Exercise illustrations: Karen Kuchar
Other illustrations: Margaret Pesek, www.designmunkee.com

Library of Congress Cataloging-in-Publication Data

Six weeks to losing it for good / edited by Emily Lapkin, with Liz Neporent, and Lynn Grieger.
    p. cm.
  ISBN 1-4016-0096-4 (pbk.)
  1. Weight loss. 2. Women—Health and hygiene. I. Lapkin, Emily. II.
Neporent, Liz. III. Grieger, Lynn.
  RM222.2.S5595 2003
  613.7'045—dc21

                           2003005931

Printed in the United States of America
03 04 05 06 07 — 5 4 3 2 1

6 weeks to

LOSING IT FOR GOOD

CANCELLED

Other Books from iVillage Solutions

CONTENTS

6 *weeks to*

LOSING IT FOR GOOD

WHAT'S DIFFERENT ABOUT THIS DIET?

More than 32,000 women lost thousands of pounds while participating in iVillage's Lose It for Good Community Challenge®. This book provides you with the tools to follow that plan.

iVillage, a leading women's website, provides information and support to women on a wide range of topics. It has always been our mission to provide solutions to the problems you most need help with. And as women, we know that losing weight and keeping it off is near the top of that list, so we've been offering expert-based diet and fitness advice since 1996. In the fall of 2000, we decided to take our diet and fitness programming one step further. We surveyed more than 3,000 women about their diet and fitness habits to uncover the biggest hurdles women face in achieving long-term weight loss success. We confirmed many of our hunches—and discovered a few things that surprised us.

Among other things, women told us:

- The number one reason they can't lose weight is not having the time to exercise or prepare special meals.
- Nearly 40 percent of them skip one meal a day.
- One-third say that eating fast food is their biggest "diet buster."

- More than half are not exercising regularly, and almost three-fourths cite lack of motivation for the reason.
- Those who do exercise prefer simple activities such as walking and using cardio machines, including treadmills, elliptical trainers, and stationary bicycles.
- They are most likely to give in to cravings at night and on the weekends.

With experts Lynn Grieger, a registered dietitian and certified diabetes educator, and Liz Neporent, an exercise physiologist, we took those survey responses and set out to create a weight loss program that would give women a realistic way to shed unwanted pounds—and that didn't presume "one size fits all" when it comes to eating and exercise.

The result was The Lose It for Good Community Challenge—a six-week online program offering flexible, customized diet and fitness routines designed to help women lose weight by addressing the very issues that hindered them most.

Because women told us their cravings often drove them to ditch their diets, we created a meal plan that worked to curb cravings by offering small portions of favorite treats. Because many women said they couldn't stick with an exercise routine due to lack of money or lack of time to visit a gym, we developed a workout regimen that could be done with no gym membership or special equipment whatsoever.

The program ran on iVillage during January and February 2001 and the results were amazing. More than 32,000 women signed up, and those who tracked their weight loss with our interactive tools reported dropping nearly *7,000 pounds*—and 3,500 inches. Participants loved the flexibility, the fact that the menus featured "yummy" foods such as grilled cheese sandwiches and chocolate pudding, and the way the pounds kept coming off, week after week. It was a program women finally felt they could stick with—and that's why we decided to share it with you!

We adapted that same plan into this book—which you can carry with you wherever you go, and to places where a computer can't go. It will tuck easily into your briefcase, gym bag, or carry-on bag.

Think of this book as your personal diet buddy. Not only does it include weekly diet and exercise plans designed just for you, but it also offers daily inspirational tips, hints for better workouts, nutrition and fitness advice from leading experts, observations from women who followed the plan, and spaces for you to keep track of your moods and eating and exercise habits.

In a crisis, read a daily tip or share an experience of a diet companion. Write down your feelings. Make this book your genuine secret weapon that provides the tools you need to reach your goals.

For additional support when you are near a computer with online access, you can visit the Losing it for Good message board at iVillage (www.ivillage.com/lifg). There you can speak with other dieters on this program who know what you're going through at any hour, day or night.

Congratulations on taking the first step to a fitter and healthier you!

Emily Lapkin
Director, iVillage Diet, Fitness, and Health

HOW TO USE THIS BOOK

Six Weeks to Losing It for Good is built around the premise that no one diet or exercise program fits every woman's needs. So we've designed multiple eating and workout plans. To help you identify which ones are right for *you*, we've developed diet and fitness personality quizzes that will tell you the menu plan and fitness routine that specifically suit your lifestyle. You'll also find special areas for journaling, plenty of inspirational tips, recipes, how-to instruction for at-home exercises—in short, everything you need to make this work for you.

Here, step by step, is how you will use the materials in this book.

Step 1: Make the commitment. Fill out the Commitment Contract that you'll find immediately after this section. The Commitment Contract is your promise to yourself that you'll make your best effort to stick with this program and see it through. You can keep this page in this book, or remove it and hang it up where it can remind you of your goals when temptation looms: on the refrigerator door, the snack cabinet, your bedroom mirror.

Step 2: Identify your issues. Take the "What's Your Diet Personality?" assessment on page 9 and "What's Your Fitness Personality?" assessment on page 12. These simple quizzes, designed by experts, will help determine which particular diet plan and fitness routine will help you overcome your weight loss obstacles.

Sign on for Daily Support

For day-to-day support, join fellow readers on the Losing It for Good message board on iVillage.com at www.ivillage.com/lifg. (If you don't have Internet access at home, you can sign on at your local library.) Here you can find inspiration, answers, and encouragement from women following the same program as you.

Step 3: Take your measurements. After you determine the optimum regimen for yourself, you will record your baseline measurements in the space provided. (Don't worry—our step-by-step guide makes this part easy to do and foolproof!) Knowing exactly where you've started will help you see just how far you've come each week.

Step 4: Begin your program. Follow your particular program each week, using the menus and workout plans provided. You'll find expert answers to common fitness and nutrition questions relevant to your program throughout. It's important to not feel like you're going it alone, so you can follow the weekly ups and downs of two women, Kim and Martha, "Your Diet Companions," who participated in the original Lose It for Good Community Challenge. You'll also find many questions and answers from original participants, which will be helpful throughout the weeks ahead.

Step 5: Start your journal. We've provided a journaling section for each of the six weeks. Each day record what you've eaten (especially if you've slipped a bit!), what you did for exercise, what your mood was like, and what issues arose during the day. Keeping track of your efforts will help keep you inspired *and* make you aware of both good and bad habits. You'll also find a daily "Pep Talk" at the start of each day's journal section. These inspiring quotes are from noted psychologist Ann Kearney-Cooke, Ph.D., and from members of iVillage who participated in the original Community Challenge. If you have other favorite motivational quotes, add them to your daily journal.

Step 6: Measure your progress. At the end of each week's journaling section, there's a space to enter your weekly measurements. Don't get discouraged, and don't skip these—even if you think you're not going to like what you see. Having a clear understanding of your progress will help you stay (or get back) on track.

We know that most weight loss goals can't be reached in six short weeks. That's why these plans were designed to be safe and healthy for long-term use. If you have more to lose, simply continue with your meal plan and exercise routine. And continue monitoring your progress in a journal of your own. Remember, you can find support at any hour on the Losing it for Good message board at iVillage (www.ivillage.com/lifg).

And when you *do* reach your weight loss goals, realize that if you return to your previous eating habits, you will slowly but surely regain the weight you lost. Continue with your exercise program, change it, or expand on it. Vary your meals gradually at first, and monitor your weight so it doesn't start creeping back on.

Now that you know how the program works, it's time to start Losing It for Good!

MY COMMITMENT CONTRACT

I, _____, promise myself that I will make my best effort to follow this book's diet and fitness routines as directed.

I, _____, promise myself that I will ask my family, friends, and coworkers to be supportive of my efforts.

I, _____, understand that I am not alone in this effort and will read the tips and encouragement in the book and keep my daily journal. If possible, I will visit the iVillage Lose It for Good message board (www.ivillage.com/lifg) to meet other women on the program and share tips and advice.

I, _____, promise myself that I will not give up if and when I encounter temporary setbacks, and I promise to renew my commitment to the program the following day.

Signed _____

Date _____

Please note: Before beginning this or any other diet and exercise program, consult with your personal physician.

MEET YOUR DIET DREAM TEAM

Two experts in nutrition and fitness developed the eating and exercise plans and information for *Six Weeks to Losing It for Good* and the online Lose It for Good Community Challenge. Together, they've helped hundreds of thousands of women on iVillage to lose weight and follow more healthful lifestyles. Now they bring their expertise to you.

Liz Neporent, who developed the fitness philosophies and plans for this book, has been in the fitness field for more than 18 years. She has a master's degree in exercise physiology and is certified by the American College of Sports Medicine, the American Council on Exercise, and the National Strength and Conditioning Association. Liz has been the fitness expert on iVillage for more than six years, and writes a regular weekly column on fitness issues and trends.

She is currently on the board of directors and board of advisors of the American Council on Exercise. She cowrote *Fitness for Dummies* and *Weight Training for Dummies* and wrote *Fitness Walking for Dummies.* She is also author of *The Ultimate Body: 10 Perfect Workouts for Women,* which addresses common fitness challenges such as weight loss, how to begin, and how to sculpt great legs.

Liz writes and is frequently quoted in many publications, including the *New York Times, Newsday, Fitness Magazine,* and *Family Circle.* When Liz isn't writing about health, fitness, and science, she is the creative director for Plus One Fitness, a fitness center management and consulting company based in New York City.

Lynn Grieger developed the diet philosophy and meal plans featured in this book. A registered dietitian and certified diabetes educator, Lynn teaches college-level nutrition courses and works with private clients on healthy nutrition and weight loss. She consults with community groups and schools to promote healthy eating habits. Lynn says, "I believe that eating a healthy, well-balanced diet is key not only to long-term health and weight control, but also is important in a busy and active life."

Lynn has been the healthy eating expert on iVillage for more than six years, and writes a regular weekly column covering a vast array of nutrition issues and evaluating the latest weight loss trends.

WHAT'S YOUR DIET PERSONALITY?

The Losing It for Good program offers two different diet plans designed to help you overcome specific weight loss challenges. To find the program that's best for you, take this simple assessment.

Complete each sentence with the statement that best describes your eating habits and opinions about dieting.

1. You eat
    a. at traditional mealtimes
    b. whenever cravings strike

2. You skip meals
    a. sometimes
    b. very frequently

3. When breakfast rolls around, you're likely to
    a. eat whatever the rest of your family is eating
    b. skip it (that is, until you indulge in your favorite mid-morning snack)

4. In the afternoons you usually
    a. feel stuffed and sleepy from eating such a big lunch
    b. snack constantly, because you're always hungry

5. At dinner time you
   a. prepare something quick and convenient (though not necessarily healthy) that the family enjoys
   b. have a bite of this, a bite of that, followed by your favorite TV snacks

6. You snack
   a. occasionally on whatever happens to be around
   b. almost all the time—sometimes you'll make a special trip to the store to get what you're craving

7. You probably weigh more than you'd like to because
   a. you regularly eat the same fattening foods your friends and family love
   b. you can't stop eating cookies, candy, chips, or any other treat that crosses your path

8. You'd finally lose weight if you
   a. had the time to prepare healthier meals
   b. could get yourself to stop snacking

9. Your ideal diet would include
   a. plenty of easy-to-prepare meals that won't pack on pounds
   b. plenty of satisfying and healthy snacks

Add up the number of As and Bs you chose. Find the category in which you had the most responses to determine your diet personality.

Mostly As: *No Time to Diet*

If you chose mostly As, our *No Time to Diet* meal plan is just for you. Your busy schedule means you're grabbing food you can eat on your way out the door or in the car, or something you can toss in the microwave and eat quickly. You're not alone in your habit of eating on the run—38 percent of women we surveyed eat prepared or prepackaged foods three to five times a week. We have included plenty of healthy fast-food meals for those times when the only food source in sight is a drive-through, and we've designed the rest of this plan around meals you can make in 30 minutes or less. Each basic menu provides between 1,500 and 1,700 calories per day.

Mostly Bs: *Conquer Your Cravings*

We designed our *Conquer Your Cravings* eating plan just for you. This plan will help you eat sensibly yet still enjoy your favorite treats, and supplies three meals and three snacks every day. Because our survey told us that 53 percent of women tend to give in to their cravings in the evenings, we've designated one snack as an after-dinner treat. But don't ignore portion sizes—measure out a serving rather than eating out of the bag or box. Each of the basic menus provides between 1,500 and 1,700 calories (most snacks included). For snacking emergencies, we provide one additional low-calorie snack suggestion that isn't included in the total calorie count.

WHAT'S YOUR FITNESS PERSONALITY?

The Losing It for Good program offers three individualized fitness programs designed to fit different lifestyles and help overcome issues that may have made you an "exercise dropout" in the past. To find the plan that's best for you, take this assessment.

Complete each sentence with the statement that most accurately describes your exercise habits and opinions about fitness.

1. When you exercise, you tend to work out
   a. when it's fairly easy and convenient to do so
   b. until you get bored (which happens pretty easily)
   c. long and hard (anything to get a better body)

2. In the past you've been most likely to quit exercising when
   a. you couldn't find the time to work out
   b. your workout routine got too monotonous
   c. you couldn't see any noticeable changes in your body

3. Walking is
   a. the most convenient, inexpensive form of exercise
   b. really dull, unless you have rugged terrain and fantastic scenery
   c. not enough of a workout to give you the body you want

4. Gyms are
   a. generally too expensive, and if they're far away, you'll never go
   b. good for variety if they offer lots of different cardio equipment and fun classes
   c. great for intensive classes and training

5. It's great when you've been working out for a while and
   a. you realize it's been a long time since you skipped exercising
   b. you discover a hot new aerobics class with a really motivating instructor
   c. you notice that your muscles have become more well defined

6. One of your fondest fitness memories is
   a. the job that required so much walking around, you didn't need additional exercise
   b. phys ed class, where you tried a new activity almost every day
   c. the day you discovered that you'd lost a few inches (and dimples) from your thighs

7. Your fitness hero is
   a. a woman who has been walking daily in all kinds of weather for the past 30 years
   b. a woman who takes up a new sport or workout routine every few months
   c. a woman who completely changed the shape of her body through her commitment to exercise

8. If you were to receive a fitness-related gift, you'd be happiest to get
   a. a comfortable new pair of walking shoes
   b. a month's supply of fitness videos (so no two days have to be alike)
   c. a free personal training session with a celebrity fitness pro

9. You feel most comfortable
   a. doing basic exercise, such as walking and stretching
   b. trying new activities and learning new ways to stay in shape
   c. mastering the workout that will bring you closest to your goal

10. Your ideal workout would include
    a. a simple, easy-to-follow routine
    b. lots of variety to keep you motivated
    c. the most effective training techniques

Add up the number of As, Bs, and Cs you chose. Find the category in which you had the most responses to determine your fitness personality.

Mostly As: *Simplicity Rules*

Your results show that a too-busy schedule or tight budget is likely getting in the way of your exercise plans. You need a workout routine that's flexible, simple, and convenient—and we designed *Simplicity Rules* just for you. Don't worry about committing an hour a day to the gym; this fitness plan is designed to work for women without the time or money for gyms or at-home equipment. And you'll see results!

The basic workout involves 30 to 45 minutes of aerobics or strength training, broken into short intervals throughout the day, five days a week. Walking and jogging are your best bets for aerobic activity, because they don't require a lot of fancy equipment and you can do them just about anywhere. Exercise videos are also a great choice for you. They're inexpensive and can also be found at your local library.

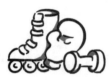

Mostly Bs: *Motivating Moves*

Your responses indicate that boredom is a big hurdle to overcome when it comes to exercise, so we've designed the *Motivating Moves* program for you. This program emphasizes fun and variety to help keep you in the game for the long haul.

The basic workout involves 30 to 45 minutes of aerobics or strength training, five days a week. You'll love energetic group classes such as step aerobics, Spinning, kickboxing, Pilates, yoga, or low-impact aerobics. If you prefer to go it alone or don't belong to a gym, try hiking, inline skating, rock climbing, horseback riding—the key is to stick with activities that are as fun as they are good for you.

Mostly Cs: *Revved-Up Results*

Your answers indicate that you may often get discouraged and abandon your exercise routine because it takes too long to see improvements. *Revved-Up Results* is the program for you. While no fitness program can change your body overnight, this plan is designed to deliver results fast.

The basic workout involves 30 to 60 minutes of aerobics or strength training, five days a week. For maximum impact, you should try high-calorie-burning activities that involve several muscle groups such as jogging, fast walking, hill walking, elliptical training, hiking, inline skating, kickboxing, Spinning, step, cross-country skiing, and jumping rope.

MEET YOUR DIET COMPANIONS

More than 32,000 women took part in the Lose It for Good Community Challenge. Many of them participated in our online support groups, sharing their ups, downs, challenges, and successes along the way. Several women in particular—our Diet Companions—kept weekly diaries and displayed them on the iVillage website. They had very different lifestyles and weight-loss issues, and helped other women see that they were not alone as they dealt with the everyday challenges of changing their eating and exercise habits. In this book, you'll find your Diet Companions' weekly entries at the end of each week's journal and tips section. Here they introduce themselves. (Their names have been changed to protect their privacy.)

Meet Kim

Kim is a 30-something mother of four children, all under the age of 10. She lives on a dairy farm in rural upstate New York with Fred, her husband of 12 years.

Weight-loss history: "I was never a small girl—at just shy of 5 feet 10 and rather big-boned, I am anything but petite," says Kim. "When I was 16, I was seriously injured and spent quite a bit of time in bed. That is when the weight began to creep on. But I wasn't really obese until after I started having kids. I gained around 25 to 35 pounds with each pregnancy. At my heaviest I was 250 pounds—that was last year. I was depressed about it and decided to change any way I could. I had several fits and starts and ended up on the Atkins diet for about six months. I lost some weight, and I went down a few dress sizes too, but I am still a snug size 18."

Biggest obstacles: Her number one obstacle is "all the yummy stuff" she keeps around for her husband and kids. "I love to bake, cook, and *sample!*" she says. Unfortunately, she *doesn't* love working out. "I also have the tendency to sabotage myself just as I am making progress and I have no clue why," she says. "I guess that is something I have to work on."

Why she wants to lose it for good: "The real reason I want to lose it for good is to feel better about myself," Kim explains. "I want to look in the mirror and say, 'boy, you look great' instead of 'boy, you need a girdle!' I want to shop in any store I want and not buy plus, queen, or extra anything. I want to be healthy. I want to be strong physically. I want to head off future troubles from my old knee injury, and from diabetes, high blood pressure, and breast cancer (all of which run in my family). I want to have more pep and energy."

Her goal: Kim wants to gain a better understanding of how to lose weight and get fit. She adds, "I am also looking to lose both inches and pounds and firm up my 'baby belly.'"

Meet Martha

Martha is a 60-something homemaker who enjoys selling on eBay. She lives with her husband and two Maltese, Sassy and Benji, in a Texas suburb. Her four children are grown and she and her husband enjoy being grandparents. She is webmaster for a large national organization. In her spare time, she dabbles in politics and genealogy, and enjoys reading, sewing, and needlework.

Weight-loss history: "What haven't I tried besides sewing up my lips?" she asks. "I've been on multiple commercial weight-loss plans—one of them over three dozen times. Counting calories, though I hate the detail, seems to work the best for me. Recording what I eat also helps."

Biggest obstacles: First, Martha hates exercise. "There is no physical activity I find appealing, though my husband and I square dance on occasion," she explains. "Also, I am diabetic and find it very difficult at this time in my life to lose weight. At the same time, I have a healthy appetite and resent very much feeling deprived on a low-calorie diet. I grew up in a very large family, where there was not enough food to go around, so deprivation is an issue with me, I think. And as a lifelong dieter, I overdosed on salad veggies years ago."

Why she wants to lose it for good: "I'm sick of being fat and ridiculed!" she says. "I'm tired of feeling 'different.'"

Her goal: She wants a plan that will let her lose two pounds a week. "My diabetes is not severe yet and I feel if I can get my weight under control, there will be less possibility of complications," she says. "Diabetes is a cruel disease and I don't want to have to deal with its effects."

TAKING MEASURE

Taking weekly measurements with a tape measure will help you keep track of your changing body. With regular exercise, your body will begin to burn fat and build muscle. Your body will be getting leaner and trimmer, although because muscle weighs more than fat, your weight may not change immediately. Or, after initially losing some weight, you may plateau for a while. Keeping a log of your measurements will remind you that your body is getting firmer and more shapely as you stick with the program—no matter what the scale says!

Here's how to do it: Find a flexible tape measure (the dressmaker's variety—not the kind you find in a hardware store) and a friend, if you want someone to help hold it around your body. Remember, never pull the tape measure so tight that it squeezes into you. It should be taut yet comfortable for the most accurate results.

Bust: Place the tape measure around your breasts and back at the fullest point (usually at the nipple line).

Waist: Place the tape measure around your midsection at the point where your waist is the smallest. If you have no natural indentation, place it at your navel line.

Hips: Place the tape measure around your body where your hips are widest. If you are pear shaped, this may be around the tops of your thighs. If your hips are narrow, measure at the top of your hipbone.

Arms: Place the tape measure around the fullest part of your arms above the elbows.

Thighs: Place the tape measure around the fullest part of your thighs. Usually this is right at the top, closest to your groin.

Now record your starting measurements on the next page.

Today's Date

Weight			
Dress size			
Pants size			
Blouse size			
Bust (inches)			
Waist (inches)			
Hips (inches)			
Arms (inches)			
Thighs (inches)			

YOUR MEAL PLANS

In this chapter you will find the meal plans for each of the six weeks of the program, with the *Conquer Your Cravings* menu plans listed first, then the *No Time to Diet* menu plans. Following these is the special *Jump Start Your Diet* plan. After Week Four, if you feel you need a "jump start" or if you have hit a plateau in weight loss, you can substitute this for one or two weeks of the program. You will find recipes immediately following the meal plans.

In the journaling sections beginning on page 125, you'll be directed to the menu to follow for each week, and you'll also find this information at the top of each menu. You may want to photocopy your particular meal plans and keep one copy in your kitchen and one at work or in your briefcase.

Vegetarians: Yes, you can follow this diet plan.

While the menus in this book include meat, eggs, and other forms of animal protein, you can follow these diet programs by making a few simple substitutions. Replace animal proteins with meatless equivalents (such as a veggie or soy burger instead of a hamburger, soy sausage instead of meat sausage, and so on) or use either tofu or legumes. In general, half a cup of cooked legumes or tofu is equal to one ounce of animal protein. You can also use egg substitutes instead of eggs, and soy milk, cheese, and yogurt instead of dairy products.

HEALTHY EATING HABITS

Following these basic principles can make any diet easier by making you feel fuller and more satisfied.

- Drink eight ounces of water with every meal and snack—a total of 64 ounces each day (more if you're exercising).
- Take a daily multivitamin or mineral supplement and an additional 500 milligrams of calcium.
- Don't rely on caffeine for energy—it may increase hunger.
- Avoid alcohol, which is high in calories and can trigger cravings.
- Measure portion sizes.
- Have healthy snacks handy to avoid impulsive eating of junk food.
- Whenever possible, sit down, relax and enjoy your food—whether it's a meal or snack—without such distractions as TV.

Smart Food Choices

These menus are guidelines. If there is a meal or set of meals you don't care for, look at the meal recommendations on another day that week and stick with those options for a while. As long as you come close to the guidelines and follow your exercise routine, you should lose weight.

Dry cereal choices: Look for high-fiber, low-fat, unsweetened cereals such as Kellogg's Special K, Post Bran Flakes, Fiber One, Wheat Chex, or Kashi Go Lean.

Fruit choices: We list a variety of fruits. As all may not be available fresh in your area (or if you don't care for a particular type), you may exchange any fruit listed for a serving of another of your favorites. In general, one serving equals one medium piece of fresh fruit (about the size of a tennis ball), ½ cup chopped, cooked, or canned fruit, or ¼ cup dried fruit.

Protein bar choices: Look for a bar with 220 to 300 calories, 10 to 20 grams protein, 30 to 40 grams carbohydrates, and 4 to 8 grams fat. Some products to look for: Balance Bar Gold, Cliff bars, Kashi Go Lean bars, Promax bars, and Revival Soy bars.

CONQUER YOUR CRAVINGS

Temptation is everywhere, and that makes dieting especially difficult for you. This plan will help you eat sensibly without giving up all your favorite treats. Your daily menu will provide between 1,500 and 1,700 calories, including a nighttime snack to keep you satisfied when you're most likely to succumb. Each day you'll also get an additional smart snacking suggestion for emergencies (not included in the total calorie count). After six weeks, you'll know the healthiest ways to curb your cravings and find the flavor you're after without getting fat.

CONQUER YOUR CRAVINGS *(PLAN A)*
(Weeks One, Three, and Five)

Day 1

Meal	What to Eat
Breakfast	1 cup oatmeal topped with ½ cup peaches 1 cup skim milk
Morning Snack	1 hard-boiled egg 1 orange
Lunch	1 cup lentil soup 1 cup cherry tomatoes 1 cup low-fat cottage cheese with pineapple
After-Work Snack	1 low-fat string cheese 4 whole-grain crackers
Dinner	3 ounces steak strips stir-fried with ½ cup red bell peppers ½ cup brown rice 1 cup steamed broccoli topped with 1 teaspoon margarine and 1 teaspoon slivered almonds 1 cup skim milk
Evening Treat	1 cup flavored decaffeinated coffee 2 gingersnap cookies
When You Just Have to Snack . . .	1 cup air-popped popcorn topped with 1 teaspoon grated Parmesan cheese has plenty of flavor but only 25 calories.

CONQUER YOUR CRAVINGS *(PLAN A)*
(Weeks One, Three, and Five)

Meal	What to Eat
Breakfast	1 cup dry cereal with 1 cup skim milk 1 cup blueberries
Morning Snack	½ cup grapes 8 whole-grain crackers with 2 tablespoons hummus
Lunch	1 grilled cheese sandwich ½ cup cherry tomatoes 1 cup fat-free yogurt
After-Work Snack	5 baked tortilla chips with ¼ cup salsa 1 cup skim milk
Dinner	2 Chicken Saté with Peanut Butter Sauce (page 76) ½ cup rice noodles 4 baby carrots ½ cup green bell pepper strips
Evening Treat	½ cup fat-free ice cream
When You Just Have to Snack . . .	Cherry tomatoes have only 4 calories each; put a handful in a bowl and enjoy.

Day 2

CONQUER YOUR CRAVINGS *(PLAN A)*
(Weeks One, Three, and Five)

Meal	What to Eat
Breakfast	1 toaster waffle with 1 tablespoon peanut butter 1 cup skim milk
Morning Snack	1 cup low-fat cottage cheese with ½ banana

Lunch	Sandwich with 2 ounces roast beef on crusty roll
	  with lettuce, tomato, and mustard
	½ cup mixed raw vegetables with 2 teaspoons
	  low-fat dressing

After-Work Snack	1 whole-wheat English muffin with 1 ounce
	  low-fat cheddar cheese melted on top
	1 cup blueberries (if fresh blueberries aren't
	  available, try frozen blueberries)

Dinner	3 ounces meat loaf
	½ cup mashed potatoes made with skim milk
	½ cup steamed carrots
	1 cup fresh baby spinach tossed with 1 teaspoon
	  olive oil, ½ teaspoon balsamic vinegar,
	  and ½ teaspoon chopped walnuts

Evening Treat	1 baked apple, filled with raisins, cinnamon, and brown sugar
When You Just Have to Snack . . .	1 cup puffed rice cereal has only 50 calories; pour yourself a bowl and munch away.

CONQUER YOUR CRAVINGS *(PLAN A)*
(Weeks One, Three, and Five)

Meal	What to Eat
Breakfast	1 cup dry cereal with 1 cup skim milk 1 slice whole-wheat toast with 1 tablespoon peanut butter 6 ounces orange juice
Morning Snack	2 tablespoons cashews mixed with 2 tablespoons dried cranberries
Lunch	Salad with 2 ounces sliced chicken breast and 1 tablespoon fat-free Caesar dressing and 1 teaspoon grated Parmesan cheese 2 Hershey Kisses
After-Work Snack	Shaky C's (page 83)
Dinner	Grilled pork chop Baked sweet potato with 1 teaspoon margarine Steamed asparagus sprinkled with 1 teaspoon Parmesan cheese and minced garlic 5 celery sticks with fat-free creamy garlic dressing
Evening Treat	Chamomile tea Butterscotch pudding
When You Just Have to Snack . . .	Sugar-free Jell-O has only 10 calories per cup— eat slowly and savor the flavor.

Day 4

CONQUER YOUR CRAVINGS *(PLAN A)*
(Weeks One, Three, and Five)

Meal	What to Eat
Breakfast	McDonalds Egg McMuffin 1 cup 1% low-fat milk
Morning Snack	1 sliced apple with 1 tablespoon peanut butter
Lunch	Sandwich wrap: Roll 2 ounces sliced, grilled or roasted chicken, 2 tablespoons shredded cheese, 2 tablespoons jarred roasted red peppers, and as much shredded lettuce as you can fit into a whole-wheat wrap 1 kiwi (slice off the top and scoop out the delicious fruit with a spoon)
After-Work Snack	½ cup guacamole with 10 baked tortilla crisps
Dinner	⅓ pound baked fillet of sole with 2 teaspoons butter and lemon juice 1 cup frozen mixed vegetables, steamed ½ cup couscous (cooked in chicken broth for added flavor) with 1 teaspoon raisins and 1 teaspoon slivered almonds 1 cup skim milk
Evening Treat	Sugar-free hot chocolate
When You Just Have to Snack . . .	1 grape has only 4 calories—you'll find frozen grapes to be crisp, juicy, and completely refreshing.

Day 5

CONQUER YOUR CRAVINGS *(PLAN A)*
(Weeks One, Three, and Five)

Meal	What to Eat
Breakfast	"Fried" egg sandwich (cook one egg in the microwave or in a non-stick skillet) on 2 slices whole-wheat bread 1 cup skim milk
Morning Snack	Strawberry-Banana Smoothie (page 84)
Lunch	2 cups black bean soup Carrot and Raisin Salad (page 69)
After-Work Snack	3 stalks celery filled with 2 tablespoons peanut butter
Dinner	4 ounces blackened skirt steak (brush with melted butter and blackened steak seasoning before grilling or broiling) 2 cups tossed salad with $\frac{1}{4}$ cup avocado, 1 teaspoon olive oil, 1 teaspoon balsamic vinegar, and $\frac{1}{2}$ cup chopped tomatoes
Evening Treat	1 cup lemon tea and 2 gingersnap cookies
When You Just Have to Snack . . .	1 small pretzel thin has 11 calories—nibble a handful slowly to make them last a long time.

Day 6

CONQUER YOUR CRAVINGS *(PLAN A)*
(Weeks One, Three, and Five)

Meal	What to Eat
Breakfast	1 cup dry cereal with 1 cup skim milk 1 small banana
Morning Snack	1 cup low-fat cottage cheese with ½ cup peaches
Lunch	Subway 6-inch turkey sub on wheat bread with 1 tablespoon mayonnaise 1 orange
After-Work Snack	Protein bar
Dinner	4 ounces grilled chicken (marinate in your favorite fat-free salad dressing) ½ cup frozen winter squash 2 cups tossed salad with 2 tablespoons reduced-fat salad dressing
Evening Treat	Decaffeinated Earl Grey tea 2 Fig Newton cookies
When You Just Have to Snack . . .	1 cup sliced cucumber has only 14 calories— toss it with fat-free sour cream and some fresh dill, and your evening perks right up!

Day 7

CONQUER YOUR CRAVINGS *(PLAN B)*
(Weeks Two, Four, and Six)

Meal	What to Eat
Breakfast	"Fried" egg sandwich (cook one egg in the microwave or in a non-stick skillet and sandwich in a whole-wheat English muffin with 1 slice cheese) 1 cup skim milk
Morning Snack	1 cup grapes
Lunch	1 cup tuna mixed with 1 tablespoon low-fat mayonnaise and ¼ cup chopped tomato 2 cups tossed salad 1 slice rye bread with 1 teaspoon margarine
After-Work Snack	1 apple
Dinner	1 serving Shrimp Kabobs (page 81) ½ cup frozen stir-fry vegetables mixed with 1 teaspoon sesame oil and ½ teaspoon toasted sesame seeds 1 cup skim milk
Evening Treat	Peppermint tea ½ cup sorbet
When You Just Have to Snack . . .	1 animal cracker has only 5 calories—if you eat them slowly like most kids do (first bite off the legs, then the head . . .), you'll savor the flavor for very few calories. But don't eat the whole zoo—try to stick to a little herd of 5 or 6.

Day 1

CONQUER YOUR CRAVINGS *(PLAN B)*
(Weeks Two, Four, and Six)

Meal	What to Eat
Breakfast	1 cup plain yogurt with ½ cup pineapple and ¼ cup low-fat granola
Morning Snack	1 slice whole-wheat bread topped with 1 tablespoon peanut butter and ½ banana 1 cup skim milk
Lunch	Wendy's Grilled Chicken Salad with 1 tablespoon low-fat dressing 1 orange
After-Work Snack	¼ cup guacamole and 10 baked tortilla crisps
Dinner	Cheese Tortellini with Beans and Vegetables (page 72) ½ cup baby carrots 1 cup skim milk
Evening Treat	Iced green tea, combined with fruit juice if desired
When You Just Have to Snack . . .	The smallest oyster crackers have only 1 calorie each, making it easy to munch a handful.

CONQUER YOUR CRAVINGS *(PLAN B)*
(Weeks Two, Four, and Six)

Meal	What to Eat
Breakfast	1 cup dry cereal with 1 cup skim milk 1 cup blueberries
Morning Snack	1 ounce cheddar cheese 2 Wasa crackers
Lunch	Veggie burger sandwich on whole-wheat bun with lettuce and salsa ½ cup green bell pepper with 1 tablespoon low-fat dressing
After-Work Snack	¼ cup hummus ½ cup celery sticks
Dinner	White Bean Chili (page 73) ½ cup brown rice ½ cup cherry tomatoes 1 cup skim milk
Evening Treat	Baked Apple Snack (page 85) Decaffeinated Earl Grey tea
When You Just Have to Snack . . .	An icy-cold frozen sugar-free fruit-juice bar has less than 15 calories—see how long you can make one (or two!) last.

Day 3

CONQUER YOUR CRAVINGS (PLAN B)
(Weeks Two, Four, and Six)

Meal	What to Eat
Breakfast	1 protein bar 1 apple
Morning Snack	1 ounce turkey on 1 slice whole-wheat bread with lettuce, tomato, and mustard 1 cup skim milk
Lunch	1 cup minestrone soup Easy Radish and Cottage Cheese Salad (page 68)
After-Work Snack	½ small whole-grain bagel with 1 tablespoon apple butter 6 ounces tomato juice
Dinner	Easy Beef and Vegetable Stir-Fry (page 77) ½ cup brown rice 1 cup melon balls or cubes 1 cup skim milk
Evening Treat	½ cup chocolate pudding Chamomile tea
When You Just Have to Snack . . .	Peel and slice one jícama into very thin sticks, which you can dunk into your favorite fat-free dip for less than 50 total calories.

Day 4

CONQUER YOUR CRAVINGS *(PLAN B)*
(Weeks Two, Four, and Six)

Meal	What to Eat
Breakfast	½ cup plain oatmeal cooked with skim milk, sprinkled with cinnamon and 1 teaspoon brown sugar, and topped with ¼ cup peaches
Morning Snack	2 Wasa crackers 1 ounce cheese 6 ounces vegetable juice
Lunch	Grilled cheese sandwich ½ cup cherry tomatoes 1 cup sugar-free, fat-free yogurt (try a delicious dessert flavor such as crème caramel)
After-Work Snack	½ cup dry cereal mixed with 2 tablespoons dried pineapple pieces and 1 tablespoon cashews
Dinner	3 ounces barbecued grilled chicken (use your favorite bottled barbecue sauce) 1 cup grilled mixed vegetables (try a combination of zucchini, onion, and eggplant) brushed lightly with olive oil and seasoned with salt, pepper, and garlic 1 ear corn on the cob (or ½ cup sweet corn kernels) with 1 teaspoon margarine 1 cup skim milk
Evening Treat	Green tea 15 animal crackers
When You Just Have to Snack . . .	Spicy salsa will wake up your taste buds, and you don't need calorie-laden fried tortilla chips to enjoy this treat—use thinly sliced celery, green pepper, radishes, or zucchini for healthy "dippers."

Day 5

CONQUER YOUR CRAVINGS *(PLAN B)*
(Weeks Two, Four, and Six)

Meal	What to Eat
Breakfast	1 whole-grain toaster waffle topped with ½ cup strawberries and ½ cup vanilla fat-free, sugar-free yogurt 1 cup skim milk
Morning Snack	½ cup chick-peas (drain off as much liquid as possible) mixed with ½ cup sliced celery and 1 tablespoon shredded cheese
Lunch	2 ounces roast beef on a crusty roll with lettuce, tomato, and mustard ½ cup mixed raw vegetables with 2 teaspoons low-fat dressing ½ cup mixed fruit salad
After-Work Snack	1 hard-boiled egg mixed with ½ cup cottage cheese and ½ cup grated carrots
Dinner	1 serving Seafood Chowder (page 82) 1 slice whole-grain bread dipped in olive oil 1 cup sliced green and red bell peppers with fat-free ranch dressing ½ cup fruit sorbet
Evening Treat	1 cup flavored decaffeinated coffee 2 gingersnap cookies
When You Just Have to Snack . . .	Guess how many blueberries you can eat for 10 calories? Thirteen! So if you want a snack that's less than 100 calories, full of healthy nutrients, and absolutely scrumptious, choose 130 blueberries! (If fresh blueberries are unavailable, try frozen.)

Day 6

CONQUER YOUR CRAVINGS *(PLAN B)*
(Weeks Two, Four, and Six)

Meal	What to Eat
Breakfast	1 cup plain yogurt with 2 teaspoons wheat germ, 2 teaspoons sunflower seeds, 2 teaspoons chopped walnuts, and 2 teaspoons dried cranberries ½ grapefruit
Morning Snack	4 Triscuit crackers ¼ cup hummus 1 cup green bell pepper strips
Lunch	1 cup lentil soup ½ cup raw broccoli with 2 tablespoons low-fat dressing ½ cup banana pudding 1 cup skim milk
After-Work Snack	Strawberry Banana Smoothie (page 84)
Dinner	1 serving Salmon Steaks Alaska (page 79) ½ cup rice pilaf 1 cup steamed asparagus with ½ teaspoon olive oil and 1 teaspoon chopped walnuts 1 cup tossed salad with ½ cup chopped tomato, 2 tablespoons chopped avocado, ½ cup grated carrots, and 2 teaspoons oil and vinegar dressing
Evening Treat	Green tea 1 chocolate-covered graham cracker
When You Just Have to Snack . . .	We tend to eat less when we have to work for our food, and this snack fits the bill to a "C." Grab one bowl of sweet cherries (5 calories each) and an empty bowl for the pits.

Day 7

NO TIME TO DIET

If you find yourself grabbing something greasy whenever you're on the go, you're not alone. Eating right in a rush is one of the biggest challenges busy women like you face. This plan helps you fight the battle with easily prepared meals and surprisingly healthy fast-food options. You'll be satisfied—taking in between 1,500 and 1,700 calories per day—and your meal selection process will be simplified. After six weeks on this plan, you'll have the routine down, and you'll be able to make smarter choices on your own, no matter how hectic things get.

NO TIME TO DIET (PLAN A)
(Weeks One, Three, and Five)

Meal	What to Eat
Breakfast	½ cup instant oatmeal made with ½ cup skim milk and a banana
Lunch	Subway 6-inch ham sandwich with tomatoes, lettuce, and 1 tablespoon mayonnaise Small bag (about ¾ cup) of pretzels 1 orange
Mid-Afternoon Energy Boost	1 cup sugar-free, fat-free yogurt with 2 tablespoons wheat germ and 1 tablespoon raisins
Dinner	4 ounces broiled salmon seasoned with lemon juice and dill ½ cup cherry tomatoes with 1 tablespoon crumbled feta cheese and 1 teaspoon olive oil ½ cup seasoned lentils and spinach 1 cup skim milk ½ cup fruit cocktail

Day 1

NO TIME TO DIET *(PLAN A)*
(Weeks One, Three, and Five)

Meal	What to Eat
Breakfast	1 cup vanilla yogurt ½ cup fresh fruit ½ cup low-fat granola
Lunch	McDonald's regular hamburger McDonald's Tossed Salad with 1 tablespoon fat-free salad dressing
Mid-Afternoon Energy Boost	1 protein bar
Dinner	4 ounces chicken breast, glazed with honey mustard, seasoned with herbs and grilled or broiled ½ cup brown rice 1 cup frozen oriental vegetables, steamed ½ cup mandarin orange slices, and sliced banana

Day 2

NO TIME TO DIET *(PLAN A)*
(Weeks One, Three, and Five)

Meal	What to Eat
Breakfast	Small bagel with 2 tablespoons peanut butter 1 apple
Lunch	Veggie burger with lettuce and tomato on whole-wheat roll ½ cup raw veggies with 2 tablespoons low-fat dressing ½ cup applesauce 1 cup skim milk
Mid-Afternoon Energy Boost	¼ cup mixed nuts with 2 tablespoons dried fruit
Dinner	½ cup Spanish rice mixed with ¼ cup seasoned ground beef ½ cup steamed green beans mixed with ½ cup steamed carrots ½ cup pineapple 1 cup skim milk

NO TIME TO DIET *(PLAN A)*
(Weeks One, Three, and Five)

Meal	What to Eat
Breakfast	1 whole-wheat English muffin with 2 teaspoons margarine 1 hard-boiled egg ½ cup grapefruit sections
Lunch	Wendy's grilled chicken sandwich Wendy's side salad with 2 teaspoons fat-free dressing
Mid-Afternoon Energy Boost	½ cup low-fat cottage cheese with fruit 2 Wasa crackers

Dinner	Almost Instant Fajitas (page 75)
	½ cup sliced peaches topped with cinnamon
	    and brown sugar over 1 cup fat-free,
	    sugar-free vanilla yogurt
	1 cup skim milk

Day 4

NO TIME TO DIET *(PLAN A)*
(Weeks One, Three, and Five)

Meal	What to Eat
Breakfast	1 whole-wheat English muffin spread with 1 tablespoon peanut butter 1 plum
Lunch	2 slices cheese and veggie pizza 2 cups tossed salad with 2 tablespoons low-fat dressing and ½ cup chick-peas
Mid-Afternoon Energy Boost	1 protein bar
Dinner	Spaghetti with Clam Sauce (page 78) ½ cup French-cut green beans ½ cup melon cubes 1 cup skim milk

Day 5

NO TIME TO DIET *(PLAN A)*
(Weeks One, Three, and Five)

Meal	What to Eat
Breakfast	1 cup skim milk mixed with 1 packet Carnation Instant Breakfast ½ cup blueberries (mix with the milk and Instant Breakfast in a blender if desired)
Lunch	Taco Bell bean burrito Taco Bell Mexican rice
Mid-Afternoon Energy Boost	1 apple with 2 tablespoons peanut butter
Dinner	Omelet made with ¾ cup egg substitute, 1 cup frozen mixed vegetables, ½ cup raw spinach, and ¼ cup shredded mozzarella cheese 1 slice wheat toast with 1 teaspoon margarine 1 cup sugar-free, fat-free yogurt

Day 6

NO TIME TO DIET *(PLAN A)*
(Weeks One, Three, and Five)

Meal	What to Eat
Breakfast	1 cup dry cereal with 1 cup skim milk and 1 cup strawberries
Lunch	1 cup Vegetarian Chili (page 71) 1 slice rye bread with 2 teaspoons margarine 3 celery stalks with 2 tablespoons peanut butter 1 cup sugar-free, fat-free yogurt
Mid-Afternoon Energy Boost	½ cup cottage cheese with fruit 4 Triscuit crackers
Dinner	Green Giant Create-A-Meal with 3 ounces chicken and 2 cups vegetables ½ cup rice ½ cup mandarin orange slices with sliced bananas

Day 7

NO TIME TO DIET *(PLAN B)*
(Weeks Two, Four, and Six)

Meal	What to Eat
Breakfast	Tofu Breakfast Burrito (page 66) 1 orange

Lunch	Boston Market turkey sandwich
	    (order without cheese and sauce to
	    lower calories)
	Boston Market fruit salad
	1 cup skim milk

Mid–Afternoon Energy Boost	Nestlé Sweet Success shake

Dinner	Lemon Herb Chicken (page 74)
	½ cup brown rice pilaf with
	    1 teaspoon slivered almonds
	½ cup steamed green beans
	½ cup baby carrots
	1 cup skim milk
	1 cup fresh strawberries topped with
	    1 tablespoon fat-free whipped cream
	    (if fresh strawberries aren't available,
	    try frozen unsweetened strawberries)

Day 1

NO TIME TO DIET *(PLAN B)*
(Weeks Two, Four, and Six)

Day 2

Meal	What to Eat
Breakfast	Subway Ham and Egg Breakfast Deli Sandwich 1 cup skim milk

Lunch	3 ounces turkey breast on whole-wheat
	     pita bread with mustard, with plenty
	     of lettuce
	½ cup fruit salad

Mid-Afternoon
Energy Boost
	Trail mix on the run:
	     Mix together ½ cup Cheerios,
	     2 tablespoons almonds, and 1 tablespoon
	     raisins

Dinner	1 taco (Use the leanest ground beef you can
	     find and drain off all the fat before adding
	     the taco sauce. Soft taco shells have fewer
	     calories than the crisp shells. Pile on as
	     many vegetables as you can.)
	1 sliced kiwi
	1 cup skim milk

NO TIME TO DIET *(PLAN B)*
(Weeks Two, Four, and Six)

Meal	What to Eat
Breakfast	1 cup plain yogurt mixed with ½ cup applesauce, ½ cup dry cereal, 2 tablespoons chopped walnuts, and ½ banana
Lunch	Chinese takeout: ½ cup fried rice, 3 ounces sweet and sour pork, and 1 cup mixed vegetables 1 fortune cookie
Mid–Afternoon Energy Boost	1 protein bar 1 cup grapes
Dinner	From the grocery store or Boston Market: 3 ounces white meat rotisserie chicken ½ cup three-bean salad ½ cup steamed broccoli with 1 teaspoon margarine 1 cup skim milk ½ cup sorbet

Day 3

NO TIME TO DIET (PLAN B)
(Weeks Two, Four, and Six)

Meal	What to Eat
Breakfast	1 cup dry cereal with 1 cup skim milk ½ grapefruit
Lunch	Burger King hamburger Burger King Garden Salad with 1 tablespoon low-fat dressing
Mid–Afternoon Energy Boost	1 cup sugar-free, fat-free yogurt mixed with ¼ cup dried fruit

Dinner	Crab salad (1 cup crab meat mixed with ¼ cup
	    diced celery, 1 tablespoon diced pimento,
	    1 teaspoon lemon juice, and 1 tablespoon
	    light mayonnaise)
	1 cup mixed greens, ½ cup chopped tomatoes,
	    ½ cup chopped red bell peppers,
	    and ¼ cup diced avocado
	1 slice pumpernickel bread with
	    1 teaspoon margarine
	1 cup skim milk
	½ cup peaches

Day 4

NO TIME TO DIET (PLAN B)
(Weeks Two, Four, and Six)

Meal	What to Eat
Breakfast	1 cup plain instant oatmeal cooked with skim milk, topped with ½ cup applesauce 1 hard-boiled egg
Lunch	1 cup tuna salad with 2 cups tossed salad 1 slice rye bread with 1 teaspoon margarine 1 apple
Mid-Afternoon Energy Boost	1 cup mixed raw celery and green pepper ¼ cup hummus 1 orange
Dinner	3 ounces lean roast beef (from the deli counter) ½ cup steamed carrots ½ cup fruit cocktail 1 cup skim milk

Day 5

NO TIME TO DIET *(PLAN B)*
(Weeks Two, Four, and Six)

Meal	What to Eat
Breakfast	½ cup low-fat cottage cheese with fruit 1 whole-wheat English muffin with 2 teaspoons peanut butter 1 cup skim milk
Lunch	Wendy's small chili Wendy's Mandarin Chicken Salad
Mid-Afternoon Energy Boost	1 protein bar
Dinner	2 frozen ricotta-stuffed shells with tomato-meat sauce 1 cup steamed spinach ½ cup pineapple

Day 6

NO TIME TO DIET *(PLAN B)*
(Weeks Two, Four, and Six)

Meal	What to Eat
Breakfast	1 protein bar 1 tangerine
Lunch	Subway 6-inch Sweet Onion Chicken Teriyaki Sandwich Small bag baked potato chips
Mid-Afternoon Energy Boost	8 Triscuit crackers 1 slice reduced-fat cheddar cheese 1 cup grapes
Dinner	1 slice Pizza Hut Beef Pan Pizza with extra veggies 1 breadstick 2 cups tossed salad with 2 tablespoons low-fat dressing

Day 7

JUMP START YOUR DIET

What's most discouraging for dieters? Hitting a plateau. It's much easier to stay motivated when you see great results. If your weight loss has
slowed or you need a "jump start," use this plan for a week, then return
to your regular menus. Although this plan is low-calorie (each basic
menu provides 1,000 to 1,100 calories in three meals), you can choose
up to 200 additional calories of snacks each day to curb the munchies
and still lose weight (these snacks are listed at the end of the menu plan
on page 63). Remember to record what you eat in your Daily Journals
and to take a daily multivitamin/mineral supplement.

You can substitute this plan for one or two of the six weeks of the
Losing It for Good program. It's especially helpful if you find yourself
stalled on a plateau, or need to get back on track if you've been
derailed the previous week. It is *not* recommended that you follow this
menu plan for more than two weeks.

JUMP START YOUR DIET

Meal	What to Eat
Breakfast	1 slice whole-grain bread with 1 teaspoon margarine 1 scrambled egg 1 orange
Lunch	Salad made with 2 ounces grilled chicken, 2 cups mixed greens, ½ cup chick-peas, and 2 tablespoons oil and vinegar dressing 2 rye crackers 1 cup skim milk
Dinner	2 Shrimp Kabobs (page 81) with tomatoes, green peppers, and onions ½ cup brown rice ½ cup sautéed snow peas

Day 1

JUMP START YOUR DIET

Meal	What to Eat
Breakfast	1 cup oatmeal with ½ cup skim milk and ½ banana
Lunch	2 cups Vegetarian Chili (page 71) ½ cup low-fat cottage cheese with ¼ cup diced pineapple 4 baby carrots with 1 tablespoon low-fat ranch dressing 1 cup skim milk
Dinner	4-ounce turkey burger topped with mushrooms, lettuce, and tomato 2 cups tossed salad with 1 tablespoon fat-free dressing ½ cup mixed orange and grapefruit sections

Day 2

JUMP START YOUR DIET

Meal	What to Eat
Breakfast	Turkey Bacon Breakfast Burrito (page 65) 1 cup skim milk
Lunch	1 cup split pea soup 1 slice dark rye bread with 1 teaspoon margarine ½ cup green bell pepper strips 1 sliced apple
Dinner	3 ounces grilled sirloin, mixed with 1 cup stir-fry vegetables ½ cup rice noodles 2 cups mixed romaine lettuce, kale, and spinach with fat-free Italian dressing Poached Pears with Chocolate Sauce (page 86)

Day 3

JUMP START YOUR DIET

Meal	What to Eat
Breakfast	1 cup dry cereal with 1 cup skim milk ½ cup of your favorite berries
Lunch	Wendy's grilled chicken sandwich Wendy's side salad with 2 teaspoons fat-free dressing
Dinner	1 cup pasta with 5 small turkey meatballs (about 2 ounces) and ½ cup marinara sauce ½ cup steamed green beans 1 cup skim milk

Day 4

JUMP START YOUR DIET

Meal	What to Eat
Breakfast	1 cup dry cereal with 1 cup skim milk ½ cup of your favorite berries
Lunch	Salad made with ½ cup canned tuna (in water), fat-free mayonnaise, 2 tablespoons diced celery, 2 tablespoons diced green pepper, and ¼ cup shredded carrots for a colorful and crunchy salad 2 cups mixed salad greens 2 Wasa crackers 1 cup grapes
Dinner	3 ounces grilled chicken breast (marinate in fat-free Italian dressing for a moist and flavorful treat) 1 small baked potato with 2 tablespoons low-fat sour cream ½ cup steamed broccoli 1 cup skim milk

Day 5

JUMP START YOUR DIET

Meal	What to Eat
Breakfast	½ whole-grain bagel with 1 ounce smoked salmon ½ grapefruit 1 cup skim milk
Lunch	1 whole-grain pita filled with 2 tablespoons hummus, 2 ounces shredded chicken, and ½ cup diced tomatoes 1 cup Jícama Mango Coleslaw (page 67)
Dinner	Dijon Dilled Salmon (page 80) ½ cup steamed asparagus 1 orange 1 cup skim milk

Day 6

JUMP START YOUR DIET

Meal	What to Eat
Breakfast	½ whole-grain English muffin spread with 1 tablespoon peanut butter ½ cup sliced peaches 1 cup skim milk
Lunch	1 cup Progresso beef barley soup ½ cup cherry tomatoes ½ cup low-fat cottage cheese ½ cup pineapple
Dinner	Bean and Cheese Burritos (page 70) 2 cups tossed salad

Day7

Snack Ideas for Jump Start Your Diet

Choose up to 200 calories of snacks each day to curb the munchies and still lose weight.

25-Calorie Snacks

8 ounces low-sodium tomato juice

1 large carrot

12 pretzel sticks

1 tangerine

6 celery stalks with 1 tablespoon fat-free dressing

½ cup raw cauliflower with 2 teaspoons fat-free dressing

1 piece hard candy

2 large dill pickles

2 sugar-free Jell-O snacks

½ cup raw broccoli with 1 tablespoon fat-free ranch dressing

1 cup popcorn with 1 teaspoon grated Parmesan cheese

½ cup green bell pepper sticks with 1 tablespoon fat-free dressing

12 radishes

50-Calorie Snacks

1 large tangerine

5 animal crackers

3 fresh apricots

¼ cup low-fat cottage cheese

1 cup strawberries

½ cup romaine lettuce with 2 tablespoons fat-free salad dressing

½ cup fruit cocktail

1 cup grapes

1 cup watermelon cubes

2 apple-cinnamon mini rice cakes with 1 tablespoon low-fat cream cheese

Snack Ideas for Jump Start Your Diet (continued)

½ cup applesauce

10 cherries

1 cup popcorn with 2 teaspoons peanuts

½ mango

100-Calorie Snacks

1 rice cake with 1 tablespoon peanut butter

½ cup low-fat cottage cheese

2 ounces tuna with 3 stalks celery

½ cup bran cereal with ¼ cup skim milk

2 tablespoons cashews

½ cup three-bean salad

½ cup fat-free, sugar-free pudding

½ cup frozen fat-free yogurt

1 cup chicken-rice soup

1 ounce mozzarella cheese

1 Fudgesicle

1 slice whole-wheat toast with 1 teaspoon jam

1 Jell-O pudding snack

2 tablespoons dry-roasted peanuts

LOSING IT FOR GOOD RECIPES

Turkey Bacon Breakfast Burrito

A delicious way to introduce your family to turkey bacon.

8 slices turkey bacon
Non-fat vegetable cooking spray
$\frac{1}{4}$ cup chopped green bell pepper
$\frac{1}{4}$ cup chopped onion
1 cup egg substitute
$\frac{1}{8}$ teaspoon freshly ground black pepper
$\frac{1}{2}$ cup grated, reduced-fat cheddar cheese
4 (12-inch) flour tortillas
Salsa, optional

To microwave the bacon, arrange 4 slices on a paper plate, and cover with a paper towel. Arrange the remaining 4 slices on top of toweling, and cover with another paper towel. Microwave on high until the bacon is crisp, 7 to 8 minutes. When cool enough to handle, chop the bacon into bite-size pieces. Spray a large nonstick skillet with the vegetable spray, and set over medium–high heat. Add the green pepper and onion to the skillet, and cook, stirring occasionally, until the vegetables are tender, 3 to 4 minutes. Reduce the heat to medium, and add the egg substitute and black pepper to the vegetables in the skillet. Cook, stirring occasionally, until the eggs are almost done, 2 to 3 minutes. Remove the skillet from the heat, and stir in the cheese and bacon. Wrap the tortillas in paper towels, and microwave on high for 10 to 20 seconds. Place approximately $\frac{1}{4}$ cup of the egg mixture on the lower third of each tortilla. Roll up the tortillas and serve. Top with salsa if desired.

Makes 4 servings.

Source: National
Turkey Federation

Nutritional Information:
(without salsa)

Calories: 92
Fat: 13 g
Carbohydrates: 20 g
Protein: 3 g

Tofu Breakfast Burritos

An excellent way to use tofu that your family will love. Be sure to purchase tofu processed with calcium for extra nutritional value.

2 large eggs
$\frac{1}{4}$ pound firm tofu, crumbled
Fat-free cooking spray
$\frac{1}{2}$ teaspoon dried basil
$\frac{1}{4}$ teaspoon dried oregano
$\frac{1}{4}$ teaspoon salt
Dash of freshly ground black pepper
2 (10-inch) flour tortillas
$\frac{1}{4}$ cup crumbled feta cheese
$\frac{1}{4}$ cup grated part-skim mozzarella cheese
$\frac{1}{4}$ cup salsa

Nutritional Information:

Calories: 454
Fat: 20 g
Carbohydrates: 45 g
Protein: 24 g

In a small bowl, beat the eggs. Add the tofu, and combine by mashing the tofu with the back of a fork until the tofu is in small pieces. Spray a large nonstick skillet with the cooking spray. Over medium heat, add the egg and tofu mixture, and cook briefly, stirring lightly. Add the basil, oregano, salt, and pepper, and cook, stirring, until the egg is cooked through. Transfer to a dish. Heat the tortillas one at a time in a skillet for about 30 seconds. Transfer the tortillas to two microwave-safe plates. Place half the egg mixture in the center of each tortilla. Sprinkle each with half the crumbled feta and roll up. Top each with half the grated mozzarella cheese. Microwave for 30 seconds, or until cheese on top melts. Add the salsa to the top and serve.

Makes 2 servings.

Jícama Mango Coleslaw

This recipe is a great source of fiber (from the jícama and mango) and vitamin A. Serve it often.

3 cups shredded cabbage
1 medium jícama, peeled and shredded
1 mango, peeled, pit removed, and chopped
2 scallions, white and light green parts chopped
Juice of 1 lime

In a serving bowl, combine the cabbage, jícama, mango, and scallions. Sprinkle with the lime juice, and stir to combine.

Makes 6 servings.

Nutritional Information:

Calories: 60
Fat: 0 g
Carbohydrates: 14 g
Protein: 2 g

Easy Radish and Cottage Cheese Salad

Using low-fat cottage cheese makes this a high-protein, low-carb salad.

1 cup small-curd, 2% fat cottage cheese
5 to 7 radishes, very thinly sliced
Salt
Italian flat-leaf parsley, chopped

Nutritional Information:

Calories: 216
Fat: 4 g
Carbohydrates: 11 g
Protein: 32 g

In a bowl, combine the cottage cheese and radish slices. Season to taste with salt and parsley. Refrigerate until ready to serve. *Note:* This salad will keep in the refrigerator, covered tightly with plastic wrap, for 3 to 5 days.

Makes 1 serving.

Carrot and Raisin Salad

Serve this sweet salad at your next brunch or luncheon.

4 cups grated carrots
$\frac{1}{2}$ cup raisins
1 cup drained crushed pineapple
1 tablespoon freshly squeezed lemon juice
1 teaspoon ground cinnamon

In a large mixing bowl, combine the carrots, raisins, pineapple, lemon juice, and cinnamon. Serve immediately, or refrigerate until ready to serve.

Makes 4 servings.

Nutritional Information:

Calories: 122
Fat: 0 g
Carbohydrates: 31 g
Protein: 2 g

Bean and Cheese Burritos

This make-ahead meal is the perfect food for busy women. Prepare the night before, and refrigerate until ready to bake.

1 tablespoon olive oil
1 cup chopped onion
1 clove garlic, minced
1 (28-ounce) can chopped tomatoes
1 cup tomato sauce
1/2 can green chilies, chopped
1/2 teaspoon salt
1/2 teaspoon dried oregano
1/2 teaspoon dried basil
10 (8-inch) flour tortillas
2 (16-ounce) cans fat-free refried beans
2 cups grated cheddar cheese

Preheat the oven to 350°F. In a large skillet over medium heat, add the olive oil and onion, and cook, stirring, until softened, 3 to 5 minutes. Add the garlic, and cook, stirring, for 1 minute more. Add the tomatoes, tomato sauce, chilies, salt, oregano, and basil. Raise the heat to high, and bring the mixture to a boil. Reduce the heat to medium-low, and simmer for 15 minutes. While the tomato mixture is cooking, prepare the burritos. On each tortilla place a spoonful of refried beans and some cheese. Roll up the tortilla, and place it in an ungreased baking pan. Repeat with the remaining tortillas. Pour the tomato sauce mixture on top of the burritos, and sprinkle any leftover cheese on top. Bake 20 minutes to heat through.

Makes 10 servings.

Nutritional Information:

Calories: 365
Fat: 13 g
Carbohydrates: 47 g
Protein: 16 g

Vegetarian Chili

A great way to add fiber and vitamin C to your diet—all without meat.

2 teaspoons olive oil

1 cup chopped onion

2 cloves garlic, chopped

1 cup diced green bell pepper

1 cup diced celery

1 cup diced carrot

2 cups cooked bulgur wheat

1 (28-ounce) can puréed tomatoes

2$\frac{1}{2}$ cups drained and rinsed canned kidney beans

5 teaspoons brown sugar

1 tablespoon ground cumin

1 tablespoon dried oregano

$\frac{1}{2}$ teaspoon ground coriander

Salt

In a large saucepan over medium heat, put the olive oil and heat briefly. Add the onion, and cook, stirring, until softened, 2 to 3 minutes. Add the garlic, and cook, stirring, 1 minute more. Add the bell pepper, celery, and carrot, and cook, stirring, for 2 to 3 minutes to soften the vegetables. Add the cooked bulgur, tomatoes, kidney beans, brown sugar, cumin, oregano, coriander, and salt to taste. Cover and simmer for 20 to 30 minutes to let the flavors meld.

Makes 6 servings.

Nutritional Information:

Calories: 258
Fat: 2 g
Carbohydrates: 51 g
Protein: 11 g

Cheese Tortellini with Beans and Vegetables

Adding beans to cheese-filled pasta gives this dish a hearty flavor and a double dose of protein.

8 ounces fresh or frozen cheese tortellini
1 cup vegetable stock
1 tablespoon butter
1 medium zucchini, sliced
1 small red bell pepper, diced
2 cloves garlic, minced
1 (20-ounce) can kidney beans, drained
1 tablespoon minced fresh thyme, or $\frac{1}{2}$ tablespoon dried
3 tablespoons pine nuts
Salt and freshly ground black pepper
$\frac{1}{3}$ cup freshly grated Parmesan cheese

Nutritional Information:

Calories: 440
Fat: 15 g
Carbohydrates: 56 g
Protein: 24 g

Bring a large pot of water to a boil over high heat. Cook the tortellini according to package directions. In a large, heavy skillet over medium-high heat, heat the vegetable stock and butter to a simmer. Add the zucchini, bell pepper, and garlic to the skillet, and stir to mix. Simmer for 3 minutes. Add the beans and thyme to the skillet, and stir to mix. Simmer for 3 minutes more. Pour the vegetable stock mixture into a colander set over the sink to drain. In a serving bowl, toss the tortellini with the strained vegetables, pine nuts, salt and pepper to taste, and the grated cheese. Serve hot.

Makes 3 servings.

White Bean Chili

A delicious, warm dish on a chilly, fall day.

1 pound ground turkey
1 (16-ounce) can white kidney beans, drained
1 (15-ounce) can yellow corn with green and red peppers, drained
1 (15-ounce) can diced tomatoes with oregano and garlic
2 cups jarred salsa

In a large, nonstick skillet over medium-high heat, cook the turkey, stirring occasionally, until browned. Drain, rinse, and blot the meat with a clean kitchen towel. Return the meat to the skillet, and add the kidney beans, corn with peppers, tomatoes, and salsa. Heat thoroughly over medium-high heat, about 10 minutes.

Makes 4 servings.

Nutritional Information:

Calories: 436
Fat: 12 g
Carbohydrates: 53 g
Protein: 33 g

Lemon Herb Chicken

Lemon juice adds zip to chicken breasts.

$1/2$ cup freshly squeezed lemon juice
$1/4$ cup vegetable oil
$1/4$ cup minced, Italian flat-leaf parsley
1 teaspoon dried tarragon
2 pounds boneless, skinless chicken breasts, cut into 6 portions

Nutritional Information:

Calories: 205
Fat: 8 g
Carbohydrates: 1 g
Protein: 30 g

In a large, zipper-top, plastic bag, combine the lemon juice, vegetable oil, parsley, and tarragon. Add the chicken pieces to the marinade in the bag, seal, and refrigerate for at least 4 hours. Preheat a gas grill to medium-low, or set a broiler to high. Drain and discard the marinade. Grill or broil the chicken, turning several times during cooking, until cooked through, 10 to 15 minutes.

Makes 6 servings.

Almost Instant Fajitas

Your family will love these, and they are so easy you won't mind repeated requests.

Vegetable cooking spray
4 boneless, skinless chicken breasts, cut into strips
1 (14$\frac{1}{2}$-ounce) can diced tomatoes
1 package taco seasoning
1 red bell pepper, sliced
1 green bell pepper, sliced
$\frac{1}{2}$ cup shredded Monterey Jack cheese or cheddar cheese
6 medium flour tortillas

Spray a large skillet with the vegetable cooking spray. Add the chicken strips, and cook over medium heat until browned all over, 1 to 2 minutes. Add the tomatoes, taco seasoning, and bell peppers. Cook, stirring, until the ingredients are well mixed and the vegetables are tender, 3 to 5 minutes. Serve by layering the chicken mixture and then the cheese onto warm tortillas, and wrap.

Makes 6 servings.

Nutritional Information:

Calories: 357
Fat: 11 g
Carbohydrates: 38 g
Protein: 24 g

Chicken Saté with Peanut Butter Sauce

Serve these chicken kabobs with a crisp salad or rice noodles.

For the chicken:

3 tablespoons soy sauce

2 tablespoons vegetable oil

$\frac{1}{2}$ teaspoon curry powder

1 clove garlic, minced

1 pound boneless, skinless chicken breasts, cut into 1-inch cubes

For the sauce:

1 teaspoon vegetable oil

$\frac{1}{4}$ cup sliced scallions, white and light green parts

$\frac{1}{4}$ teaspoon crushed red pepper flakes

$\frac{1}{2}$ cup smooth peanut butter

1 cup water

1 tablespoon soy sauce

$\frac{1}{2}$ teaspoon ground ginger

To make the kabobs, combine the soy sauce, oil, curry powder, garlic, and chicken cubes in a large mixing bowl. Cover and marinate in the refrigerator for 2 hours or longer. Preheat the broiler to high. Thread the chicken cubes onto wet bamboo skewers. Broil them 6 inches from the heat, turning and basting with the remaining marinade, about 5 minutes or until done.

While the chicken is broiling, make the sauce. Heat the oil in a small skillet over medium heat for 1 minute. Add the scallions and red pepper flakes, and cook, stirring, 1 minute. Stirring constantly, add the peanut butter to the skillet. Gradually stir in the water and soy sauce. Add the ginger and stir. Bring to a boil, and cook until the mixture thickens. Serve with the chicken kabobs.

Makes 4 servings.

Nutritional Information:

Calories: 380
Fat: 23 g
Carbohydrates: 8 g
Protein: 35 g

Easy Beef and Vegetable Stir-Fry

Feel free to substitute other vegetables for the mushrooms, such as steamed broccoli, julienned carrots and zucchini, or red and green bell pepper strips. You can find the pre-cut stir-fry beef strips in the beef section at most supermarkets—it's a great timesaver.

1 tablespoon vegetable oil
1 small onion, thinly sliced
1 (8-ounce) package white or crimini mushrooms
$\frac{1}{2}$ pound beef round strips for stir-frying
3 tablespoons Kikkoman stir-fry sauce

In a large skillet over medium-high heat, heat the oil for 1 minute. Add the onion to the skillet, and cook, stirring, until softened, about 2 minutes. Add the mushrooms, and cook, stirring, until lightly browned, 3 to 4 minutes. Add the beef strips to the skillet, and cook, stirring frequently, until browned and cooked through, about 4 minutes. Add the stir-fry sauce, and cook, stirring, just until heated through, about 1 minute. Spoon the beef and vegetable mix into serving dishes, and be sure to spoon some of the sauce into each dish.

Makes 3 servings.

Nutritional Information:

Calories: 198
Fat: 9 g
Carbohydrates: 8 g
Protein: 21 g

Spaghetti with Clam Sauce

Easy and fast—and not your usual spaghetti with red sauce. Give your family a new taste while keeping your time in the kitchen to a minimum.

1 pound spaghetti

2 tablespoons vegetable oil

2 cloves garlic, minced

2 (6$\frac{1}{2}$-ounce) cans chopped clams, drained, with liquid reserved

$\frac{1}{2}$ cup chopped fresh Italian flat-leaf parsley

$\frac{1}{2}$ cup dry white wine

1 teaspoon dried basil

$\frac{1}{4}$ teaspoon white pepper

Source: National
Pasta Association

Nutritional Information:

Calories: 421
Fat: 7 g
Carbohydrates: 69 g
Protein: 17 g

Cook the pasta according to package directions and drain. In a medium skillet, heat the oil over medium heat. Add the garlic, and cook, stirring, for 1 minute. Add the reserved clam liquid and parsley to the skillet, and stir to mix. Cook, stirring, for 3 minutes. Add the clams, wine, basil, and pepper. Simmer over low heat for 5 minutes. Pour the sauce over cooked spaghetti and serve immediately.

Makes 5 servings.

Salmon Steaks Alaska

This is so simple and so delicious you will want to cook it often. If steaks are frozen, thaw in the refrigerator, or cook unthawed according to package directions.

2 tablespoons freshly squeezed lime or lemon juice
1/4 teaspoon Tabasco sauce
Non-fat cooking spray
16 ounces fresh or frozen salmon steaks about 1-inch thick

Preheat the broiler to high. In a small bowl, combine the lime or lemon juice and Tabasco. Lightly coat the broiler rack with non-fat cooking spray. Place the salmon steaks on the broiler rack in a broiler pan. Brush the citrus juice and Tabasco marinade over the steaks. Transfer the broiler pan to the broiler, and set it about 4 inches from the heat. Broil 15 minutes, or until the salmon is easily flaked with a fork.

Alternate preparation: To bake, place the salmon steaks in a greased, shallow baking dish, and brush the citrus juice and Tabasco marinade over the steaks. Bake in a preheated, 350°F oven for 25 to 30 minutes, or until the salmon can be easily flaked with a fork.

Makes 4 servings.

Nutritional Information:

Calories: 100
Fat: 22 g
Carbohydrates: 1 g
Protein: 11 g

Dijon Dilled Salmon

A great fish dish, this can be served with a green salad or asparagus for a good dinner. If fresh dill isn't available, substitute 1 teaspoon dried dill weed. To reduce the fat further, use low-fat mayonnaise instead of regular.

6 tablespoons chopped fresh dill
1/4 cup mayonnaise
2 tablespoons milk
4 teaspoons Dijon mustard
1 1/2 pounds salmon fillets
2 teaspoons olive oil
1/4 teaspoon salt
1/4 teaspoon freshly ground black pepper

Nutritional Information:

Calories: 352
Fat: 19 g
Carbohydrates: 4 g
Protein: 39 g

In a small bowl, mix together the dill, mayonnaise, milk, and mustard. Preheat the broiler to high. Remove any small bones from the salmon, and cut the fillets in half. Lightly brush the olive oil on a broiler pan and its rack, and place the fillets in the pan, laying the salmon skin-side down on the broiler rack. Brush the top of the salmon with the remaining olive oil, and sprinkle each piece with the salt and pepper. Place the broiling pan about 6 inches from the heat source and broil for 7 to 10 minutes, depending on the thickness of the salmon. The fish should be golden brown on top and flake easily when done. Serve the salmon with the reserved Dijon dill sauce.

Makes 4 servings.

Shrimp Kabobs

Shrimp kabobs are a fantastic change from grilled chicken or red meat.

6 ounces jumbo shrimp
1/3 cup Kikkoman teriyaki marinade
1 scallion, finely chopped
1 clove garlic, minced
1 teaspoon freshly grated lemon peel
1/2 cup canned chunk pineapple, with some juice from can

Preheat a gas grill to medium or a broiler set to high, whichever weather permits.

Leaving the shell on the tails, peel and devein the shrimp if needed. In a medium bowl, combine the teriyaki marinade, scallion, garlic, lemon peel, and a little pineapple juice for sweetness. Add the shrimp to the marinade mixture, and toss to coat. Place 1 pineapple chunk in the curve of each shrimp, and slide the shrimp onto a skewer. Repeat with 2 to 3 shrimp per skewer. Reserve the marinade mixture. Cook about 3 minutes on each side or until pink, brushing the marinade mixture on the shrimp while cooking.

Makes 1 serving.

Nutritional Information:

Calories: 155
Fat: 1 g
Carbohydrates: 11 g
Protein: 24 g

Seafood Chowder

This stick-to-your-ribs chowder is packed with protein and surprisingly low in fat.

1$\frac{1}{2}$ cups bottled clam juice
2 potatoes, peeled and cut into $\frac{1}{2}$-inch cubes
1 medium onion, chopped
1$\frac{1}{2}$ pounds flaked whitefish, cut into bite-size pieces
2 cups evaporated skim milk (or use less depending on how thick
    you like your chowder)
Salt
Freshly ground black pepper
Paprika

Nutritional Information:

Calories: 176
Fat: 5 g
Carbohydrates: 11 g
Protein: 20 g

In a large pot combine the clam juice, potatoes, and onion. Set over medium heat, and heat to a simmer. Reduce the heat, and simmer until the potatoes are cooked, about 10 minutes. Add the fish and skim milk. Simmer until heated through, about 10 minutes more. Season with the salt, pepper, and paprika to taste before serving.

Makes 8 servings.

Shaky C's

The "C's" are for vitamin C and calcium—and this delicious shake has both!

¹⁄₂ cup sliced strawberries
¹⁄₂ cup sliced ripe bananas
¹⁄₂ cup orange juice
¹⁄₂ cup vanilla yogurt

In a blender, combine the strawberries, bananas, orange juice, and yogurt. Blend on "whirl" until the mixture is smooth and frothy. Pour into a large glass and enjoy.

Makes 1 serving.

Nutritional Information:

Calories: 201
Fat: 5 g
Carbohydrates: 42 g
Protein: 8 g

Strawberry Banana Smoothie

This is a great source of calcium and a quick and easy snack or breakfast meal.

$^3/_4$ cup frozen, unsweetened strawberries
2 small bananas
$1^1/_2$ cups low-fat plain yogurt

Thaw the strawberries for 5 to 10 minutes in a colander over the sink. Put the strawberries, bananas, and yogurt into a blender. Blend until smooth. Serve immediately, or spoon into dishes and refrigerate until ready to serve.

Makes 4 servings.

Nutritional Information:

Calories: 122
Fat: 2 g
Carbohydrates: 23 g
Protein: 6 g

Baked Apple Snack

Your home will smell like fresh apple pie while this easy dessert is baking.

4 tart apples
$1/2$ cup raisins
4 teaspoons brown sugar
2 teaspoons cinnamon

Preheat the oven to 350°F. Line the bottom of an 8 x 8-inch baking dish with parchment paper. Wash and core each apple. Place the apples upright in the prepared baking dish. Fill the centers of the apples with raisins and brown sugar. Sprinkle the cinnamon on top. Bake for 1 hour. Serve hot.

Makes 4 servings.

Nutritional Information:

Calories: 146
Fat: 0 g
Carbohydrates: 39 g
Protein: 1 g

Poached Pears with Chocolate Sauce

The tartness of poached pears blends beautifully with the sweetness of chocolate in this low-fat dessert.

2$\frac{1}{2}$ cups water
7 tablespoons sugar
Juice and grated zest of 1 lemon
1 cinnamon stick
4 pears, halved and cored
$\frac{1}{4}$ cup store-bought chocolate sauce

In a large saucepan, combine the water, sugar, lemon juice, lemon zest, and cinnamon stick. Set over high heat, bring to a boil, and cook, stirring, until the sugar is dissolved. Remove the saucepan from the heat, and carefully add the pear halves to the boiling syrup. (Pears should be covered in liquid; if not, double the amount of poaching liquid or poach in batches.) Set the saucepan over medium-low heat, and simmer gently until the pears are almost tender, 15 to 20 minutes. Remove from the heat and let the pears cool in the liquid. (The pears will continue to cook while cooling.) Drain the pears thoroughly, and pat dry on paper towels. Arrange the pear halves on individual plates. Drizzle each pear with $\frac{1}{2}$ tablespoon chocolate sauce, and serve at room temperature.

Makes 8 servings.

Source: American
Institute for Cancer
Research

Nutritional Information:

Calories: 116
Fat: 2 g
Carbohydrates: 30 g
Protein: 1 g

YOUR FITNESS PLANS

In this chapter, you'll find all the fitness plans for your specific type of exercise personality: First the *Simplicity Rules* fitness plans, then the *Motivating Moves* fitness plans, then the *Revved-Up Results* plans. Remember, the quiz you took earlier tells you which fitness plan will work for you. The top of each plan will tell you which weeks you use that particular plan, and your journal sections, which start on page 125, also will direct you to the specific plan for each of the six weeks.

According to our online survey, 55 percent of you exercise less than once or twice a week. You'll get the best results, however, if you do cardiovascular training, strength training, and stretching three to five days a week.

EXERCISE BASICS

You may also want to refer back frequently to these exercise tips, which will make your workouts safer, more productive, and more fun.

Strength train or tone regularly. Schedule workouts two to three times a week. Do at least one exercise per workout for each muscle group. (For suggestions and how-tos on some basic strength training moves, see page 102.) Rest a day between sessions to give your muscles a chance to recover and grow stronger.

Stretch after working out. Instead of stretching before a workout, stretch *after*, when your muscles are warm and limber. Hold each stretch for about 60 seconds.

Find the right intensity. Go at your own pace, but push a little. You're at the right intensity during aerobic exercise if you can feel your heart beating and you are sweating lightly. You should be able to carry on a conversation with a workout buddy—if you can't, you're pushing too hard.

Drink lots of water. By the time you feel thirsty, you're in the early stages of dehydration, which saps your energy. Drink before, after, and during your workout.

Eat for exercise. Have a light snack before exercising (leave yourself at least 30 minutes to digest) and another light snack within the 30 minutes following your workout. This will help keep your blood sugar steady so you don't zonk out in the middle of your workout or a few hours later.

Make an appointment—with yourself. Schedule exercise times and write them down in your calendar or personal organizer. Then keep that appointment, just as you would any other important engagement.

Don't go overboard. You can't make up for years of inactivity with just one workout—but you *could* hurt yourself. Do as much as you can to start, and gradually build from there: A good rule of thumb is to increase your exercise level by no more than 10 percent per week.

CALCULATING YOUR HEART RATE

To get a more accurate reading on how hard you're working, calculate your maximum heart rate by subtracting your age from 220. Multiply that number by 0.6 and 0.85 to find the low and high ends of your target heart rate zone. You should be near the upper end of this zone at the peak of your workout.

To measure your heart rate during your workout: Place the middle and index fingers of your right hand at the base of your left wrist directly below your thumb. Press lightly until you feel the thumping of your pulse. Count how many beats you feel in six seconds and add a zero to the end—you'll have a good estimate of your heart rate.

Or you can invest in a heart rate monitor and wear it during your workouts. You'll find a selection of them at sporting goods stores, or specialty stores such as bicycle shops.

SIMPLICITY RULES

This routine is flexible, simple, and convenient.

The basic workout: 30 to 45 minutes of aerobics or strength training, broken into short intervals throughout the day, five days a week.

Smart aerobic choices: Walking and jogging are your best bets for aerobic activity, because they don't require a lot of fancy equipment and you can do them just about anywhere. Exercise videos will also be a great choice. They're inexpensive, and whenever you have a spare minute at home you can pop a tape in the VCR. You may also find some at your local library that you can check out.

Time management: You don't have to clock 30 continuous minutes in the gym to see results—you can split up your exercise to fit your schedule. You'll still get great results from splitting your workout into two to three sessions. This is also a great strategy when you're just starting to get into shape because it breaks your workouts into manageable segments. Twenty minutes can seem like forever when you're just starting out, but you *know* you can manage five or ten.

To make it even better: When you're strength training, choose exercises that do double duty. For instance, lunges work both the buttocks and thighs. Add a bicep curl as you lunge and you'll also be working your arms. Another advantage of these compound exercises is that they're a bit more challenging than the ones that isolate one muscle at a time. (For explanations on how to do these and other easy at-home muscle-builders, see page 102.)

To stay focused: Add fitness moves throughout your day. Walk around your office when you're stumped rather than sit in front of your computer. Take your dog for a longer walk than usual. Play tag with your kids. These little moves add up!

- Remember to record your activities in your Daily Journal.

- Stretch all your major muscle groups post-workout, when your muscles are warm and limber. Hold each stretch 10 to 30 seconds.

- Remember, you'll burn as many calories breaking your workouts into short sessions as you would doing it all at once. So don't let a tight schedule get you down!

- You will find a wide variety of strength training exercises (with step-by-step illustrations) to choose from, starting on page 102. Aim to target each of your muscle groups.

- If it's too cold to walk or jog outside, remember that exercise videos are just as effective.

- Don't forget to rest—we recommend one day "off" for every two or three days "on."

TIPS FOR SUCCESS

SIMPLICITY RULES *(PLAN A)*
(Weeks One, Three, and Five)

Day 1	Morning: a 15-minute brisk walk At lunch: another 15-minute brisk walk Evening: 15 minutes of strength training
Day 2	Morning: a 15-minute brisk walk At lunch: another 15-minute brisk walk Evening: another 15-minute brisk walk
Day 3	Rest
Day 4	Try a 30-minute aerobic exercise video.
Day 5	Morning: a 15-minute brisk walk At lunch: another 15-minute brisk walk Evening: 15 minutes of strength training
Day 6	Rest
Day 7	Morning: a 15-minute brisk walk At lunch: another 15-minute brisk walk Evening: another 15-minute brisk walk

SIMPLICITY RULES *(PLAN B)*
(Weeks Two, Four, and Six)

Day 1	Morning: a 15-minute jog At lunch: a 15-minute brisk walk Evening: 15 minutes of strength training
Day 2	Morning: a 15-minute jog At lunch: a 15-minute brisk walk Evening: 15 minutes of strength training
Day 3	Rest
Day 4	Try a 30-minute aerobic exercise video.
Day 5	Morning: a 15-minute jog At lunch: a 15-minute brisk walk Evening: another 15-minute brisk walk
Day 6	Morning: a 15-minute jog At lunch: a 15-minute brisk walk Evening: 15 minutes of strength training
Day 7	Rest

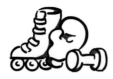

MOTIVATING MOVES

This routine emphasizes fun and variety to help keep you going.

The basic workout: 30 to 45 minutes of aerobics or strength training, five days a week.

Smart aerobic choices:
- *Adventure workouts:* Hiking, inline skating, rock climbing, horseback riding.
- *Classic workouts:* Fast walking, jogging, biking, swimming.
- *Videos or classes:* "Boot camp" training (military-style workouts with lots of calisthenics), kickboxing, low-impact or step aerobics, Pilates, Spinning, yoga.
- *Gym or home gym workouts:* Elliptical training machine, treadmill, stationary bike.

Strength training options:
- Body sculpting classes and videos.
- Weight-training circuit at the gym.
- Easy Strength Exercises on page 102—do at least one exercise for each muscle group.

Time management: Mix and match your aerobic workouts. Besides offering variety, cross training helps work several muscle groups at once, which saves time and can help prevent injury.

To make it even better: Shake up your strength-training routine. Hiring a personal trainer for even one session will teach you new tricks—and will help you perfect your technique as well. Or, take a body-sculpting class or buy a muscle-toning video to generate ideas.

To stay focused: An exercise diary can help you stick with it. Record your workouts (starting on page 126) and measurements (page 19) so you can see your progress. And take time to think about what you are trying to accomplish. When you work toward specific goals, it's easier to lace up your workout shoes each day.

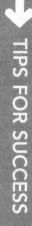

- Remember to record your activities in your Daily Journal.

- Stretch all your major muscle groups post-workout, when your muscles are warm and limber. Hold each stretch 10 to 30 seconds.

- Don't forget to rest—we recommend one day "off" for every two or three days "on."

TIPS FOR SUCCESS

MOTIVATING MOVES *(PLAN A)*
(Weeks One, Three, and Five)

Day 1	45 minutes aerobic exercise
Day 2	30 minutes strength training 15 minutes aerobic exercise
Day 3	Rest
Day 4	45 minutes aerobic exercise
Day 5	30 minutes aerobic exercise
Day 6	Rest
Day 7	15 minutes strength training 30 minutes aerobic exercise

MOTIVATING MOVES *(PLAN B)*
(Weeks Two, Four, and Six)

Day 1	45 minutes aerobic exercise
Day 2	45 minutes strength training 15 minutes aerobic exercise
Day 3	Rest
Day 4	45 minutes aerobic exercise
Day 5	30 minutes aerobic exercise
Day 6	15 minutes strength training 30 minutes aerobic exercise
Day 7	Rest

REVVED-UP RESULTS

Revved-Up Results is meant to help you see maximum results in the least amount of time, so the workouts emphasize high-intensity exercise choices that work multiple muscle groups at once. We've also included one day of interval training.

The basic workout: 60 minutes of exercise, five days a week. (If you haven't exercised in a while, start with 30-minute workouts. Extend the duration as your fitness level improves.)

Smart aerobic choices:

- *In the great outdoors:* Brisk walking, jogging, hill walking, hiking, inline skating, cross-country skiing.
- *At the gym or in your home:* Jumping rope, kickboxing, Spinning, step aerobics, or an elliptical training machine.

Strength training options:

- One circuit of strength training machines at your gym.
- Easy Strength Exercises on page 102—do at least one exercise for each muscle group.

Time management: When you work out with weights, take little or no rest before moving on to the next exercise. This keeps your heart rate up, helps strengthen your muscles, and saves time. Try alternating upper- and lower-body exercises so you don't tire out as quickly.

To make it even better: For your interval workout on Day 4, after warming up for five minutes or so, pick up the pace so you feel challenged for three minutes, then slow down to recover. Repeat this hard-easy cycle until you have completed your workout. Finish up with a nice, easy cool-down. If you're using your heart rate as a guide, you should be at the upper end of your target heart rate zone (see page 89) during the hard intervals and toward the lower end during warm-up, recovery intervals, and cool-down. You can modify any aerobic activity, such as jogging or walking, for interval training.

To stay focused: You can gauge results only when you know exactly where you started. Before you begin the plan, record your weight and measurements on page 19. Check weight and measurements throughout the program and you'll have tangible evidence of how much you're shaping up.

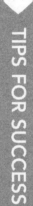

- Remember to record your activities in your Daily Journal.

- Stretch all your major muscle groups post-workout, when your muscles are warm and limber. Hold each stretch 10 to 30 seconds.

- Mix it up. You need to give your body time to recover from all of your different activities, and a varied workout schedule will help.

- Don't forget to rest—we recommend one day "off" for every two or three days "on."

TIPS FOR SUCCESS

REVVED-UP RESULTS *(PLAN A)*
(Weeks One, Three, and Five)

Day 1	45 minutes aerobic exercise 15 minutes strength training
Day 2	60 minutes aerobic exercise
Day 3	Rest
Day 4	Try this walk–jog interval program: After warming up for 5 minutes, alternate 3 minutes of moderately paced walking with 3 minutes of jogging. Do 10 interval cycles, then cool down and stretch.
Day 5	60 minutes aerobic exercise
Day 6	45 minutes aerobic exercise 15 minutes strength training
Day 7	Rest

REVVED-UP RESULTS *(PLAN B)*
(Weeks Two, Four, and Six)

Day 1	45 minutes aerobic exercise 15 minutes strength training
Day 2	45 to 60 minutes aerobic exercise
Day 3	Rest
Day 4	Fast–slow aerobic exercise interval program: After warming up for 5 minutes or so, alternate 3 minutes of moderately paced exercise with 3 minutes of slower-paced exercise (do 10 interval cycles, then cool down and stretch).
Day 5	45 to 60 minutes aerobic exercise
Day 6	45 minutes aerobic exercise 15 minutes strength training
Day 7	Rest

EASY STRENGTH EXERCISES

Here are your illustrated instructions for the exercises suggested in each of the three fitness plans.

Strength training builds lean muscle, which boosts metabolism and helps burn calories. During each exercise session, choose one move for each body part and do 15 repetitions. If you're just starting out, one set will be enough; as you improve, build to three sets. Weights should be heavy enough that you feel challenged during the last few repetitions (be sure to add weight as you get stronger). Once you get the routine down, you should be able to do one set of 15 repetitions for every part of the body in about 15 minutes.

Buttocks

Squat
(figure a)
Stand with your feet hip-width apart, your weight slightly back on your heels. Pull in your abdominals, and stand up tall with square shoulders and a lifted chest.

(figure b)
Sit back and down, as if you're sitting into a chair directly behind you. You may find it helpful to raise your arms out in front of you for balance as you move. Lower as far as you can without leaning your upper body more than a few inches forward (this depends on your flexibility and your build). If you can bend your knees far enough that your thighs are parallel to the floor, don't go any further, and don't allow your knees to travel out in front of your toes. Once you feel your upper body fold forward over your thighs, straighten your legs and stand back up. Take care not to lock your knees at the top of the movement.

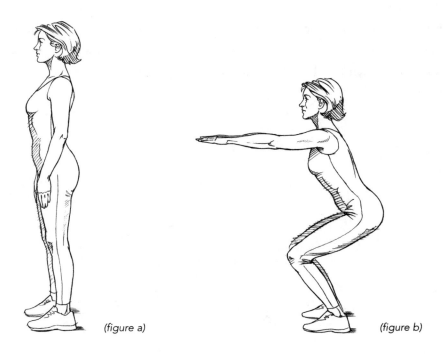

(figure a)   *(figure b)*

Glute Press

(figure a)

Kneel on your elbows and knees on top of a thick towel or exercise mat with your knees directly under your hips and your elbows under your shoulders. Clasp your hands together or turn your palms toward the floor. Flex your right foot so that your heel lifts up. Tilt your chin slightly toward your chest, and pull in your abdominals so that your back doesn't sag toward the floor.

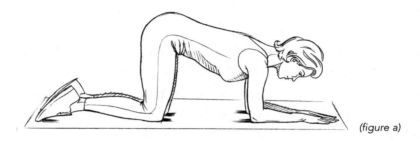

(figure a)

(figure b)

Keeping your knee bent, lift your right leg and raise your knee to hip level. Then slowly lower your leg back down. Between repetitions, your knee should almost, but not quite, touch the floor. Complete all the repetitions with one leg before switching sides.

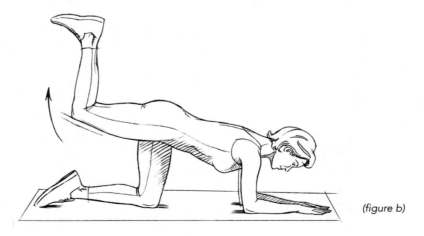

(figure b)

Front of Thighs

Alternate Lunges

(figure a)

Stand with your feet hip-width apart, with your weight back a little on your heels. Pull in your abdominals and stand up tall with square shoulders and a lifted chest.

(figure b)

Lift your right toe slightly and, leading with your right heel, step your right foot forward about a stride's length, as if you're trying to step over a crack in the sidewalk. As your foot touches the floor, bend both knees until your right thigh is parallel to the floor and your left thigh is perpendicular to it. Your left heel will lift up off the floor. Press off the ball of your foot and step back to the standing position. Do the next repetition with your left leg and continue alternating legs until you have completed the set.

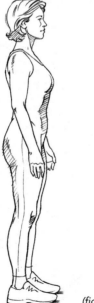

(figure a)

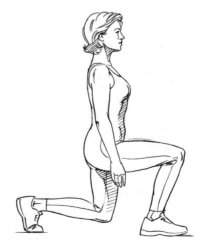

(figure b)

Straight Leg Raise

(figure a)

Sit on the floor or lean against a wall with your legs right out in front of you. (Or bend your right knee into your chest if that's more comfortable.)

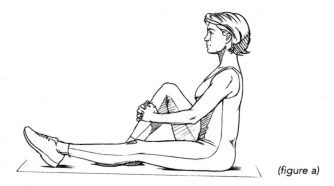

(figure a)

(figure b)

Raise your left leg a few inches. Hold for five slow counts, lower, and repeat until you complete the set. Then switch legs.

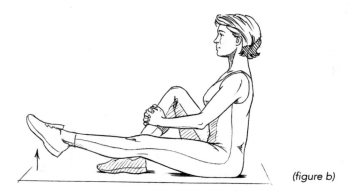

(figure b)

Stationary Lunge

(figure a)

Stand tall with your legs straddled about a stride's length apart.

(figure b)

Bend both knees until your front thigh is parallel to the floor and your back leg is perpendicular to it, with your back knee hovering just above the floor. Stand back up to the start, taking care not to lock your knees or overarch your back. Complete all reps before switching legs.

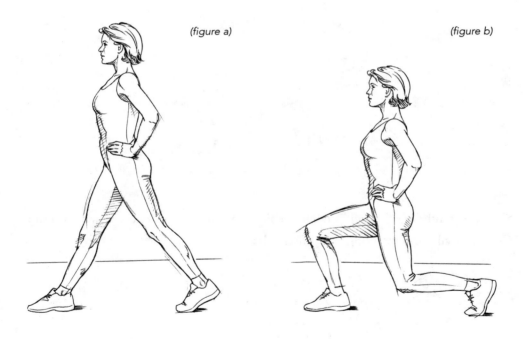

(figure a)   *(figure b)*

Back of Thighs

Kneeling Leg Curl

(figure a)

Kneel on your elbows and knees on a thick towel or exercise mat, with your knees directly under your hips and your elbows under your shoulders. Clasp your hands together or turn your palms toward the floor. Flex your right foot so that your heel lifts up. Tilt your chin slightly toward your chest, and pull in your abdominals so that your back doesn't sag toward the floor. Keeping your knee bent, lift your right leg, and raise your knee to hip level.

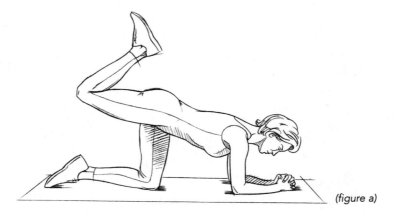

(figure a)

(figure b)

Slowly extend your leg out straight behind you and then bend it back in again. Complete all the repetitions with one leg before switching sides.

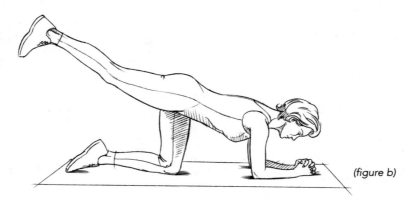

(figure b)

Leg and Back Bridge
(figure a)

Lie on your back with your knees bent and feet flat on the floor about hip-width apart. Rest your arms wherever they're most comfortable. Gently pull in your abdominals toward your spine. Don't tilt your head up and back.

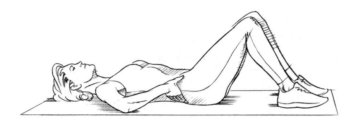

(figure a)

(figure b)

Press your feet downward, pull abdominals inward and tuck pelvis under, so that you gently lift your entire back, from the buttocks to the shoulder blades, up off the floor. Hold position for five slow counts and slowly lower back down to start.

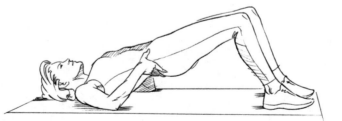

(figure b)

Calves

Toe Raise

(figure a)

Stand tall and rest your hands against a wall or a sturdy object for balance.

(figure b)

Raise up on the tips of your toes to lift your heels up off the floor. Hold the position for a moment, and then lower your heels back down.

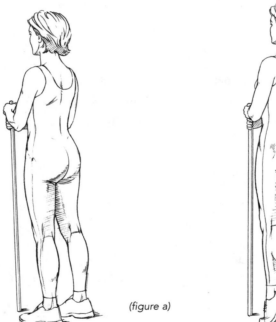
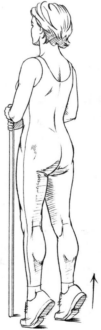

(figure a)   *(figure b)*

Toe Raise with Step

(figure a)

Stand tall on the edge of a step, with the balls of your feet on the edge. (Or, if using a step aerobics platform, place two sets of risers underneath the platform.) Rest your hands against a wall or a sturdy chair for balance.

(figure b)

Raise your heels a few inches above the step so that you're on your tiptoes. Hold the position for a moment, and then lower your heels back down so they are below the platform, to stretch your calf muscles.

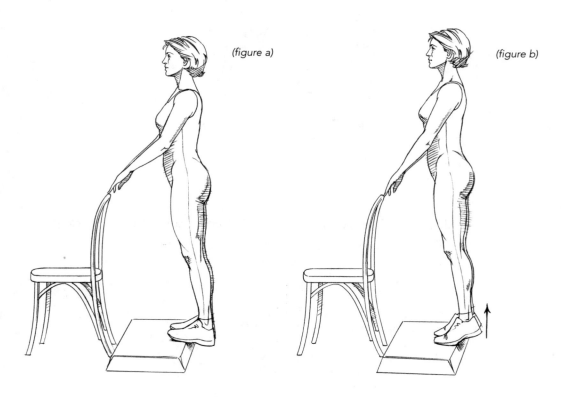

(figure a)   *(figure b)*

Chest

Push-Ups

(figure a)

Lie on your stomach, bend your knees, and keep ankles together or cross them, whichever is more comfortable for you. Bend your elbows and place your palms on the floor a little to the side and front of your shoulders. Straighten your arms and lift your body so you're balanced on your palms and knees. Tuck your chin a few inches toward your chest so your forehead faces the floor. Tighten your abdominals.

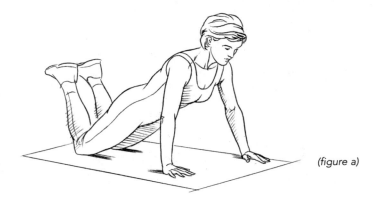

(figure a)

(figure b)

Bend your elbows and lower your entire body at once. Rather than trying to touch your chest to the floor, lower only until your upper arms are parallel to the floor. Push back up.

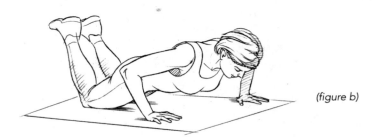

(figure b)

Dumbbell Press

(figure a)

Lie on a bench, aerobic step, or the floor with your knees bent, feet flat on the floor with a dumbbell in each hand. Push the dumbbells up so your arms are directly over your shoulders and your palms face away from you. Pull in your abdominals, but don't jam your back into the bench or floor or let it arch way up. Tilt your chin toward your chest. Lower the dumbbells down until your elbows are slightly below your shoulders.

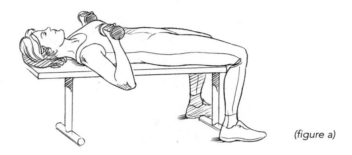

(figure a)

(figure b)

Push the weights back up, taking care not to lock your elbows or allow your shoulder blades to rise off the bench.

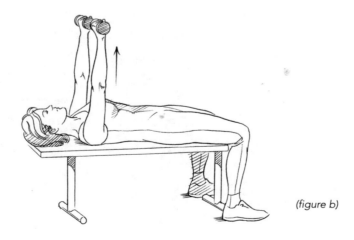

(figure b)

Fly

(figure a)

Lie on a bench, aerobic step, or the floor with your knees bent, feet flat with a dumb-bell in each hand. Push the dumbbells up so your arms are directly over your shoulders and your palms face in toward each other. Pull in your abdominals, but don't jam your back into the bench or floor or let it arch way up. Tilt your chin toward your chest.

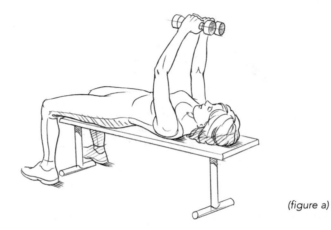

(figure a)

(figure b)

Lower the dumbbells down and out to the side until your elbows are slightly below your shoulders. Push the weights back up, taking care not to lock your elbows or allow your shoulder blades to rise off the bench.

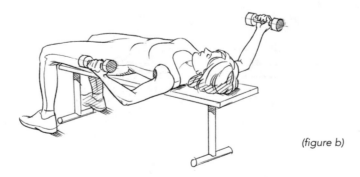

(figure b)

Back

One-Arm Row

(figure a)

Stand to the right of your weight bench or a chair and hold a dumbbell in your left hand with your palm facing in. Pull in your abdominals and bend forward from your hips so that your back is naturally arched and roughly parallel with the floor and your knees are slightly bent. Place your right hand on top of the bench for support and let your left arm hang down.

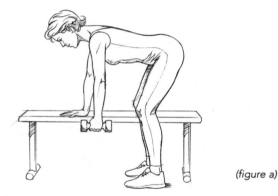

(figure a)

(figure b)

Bend your left arm up until your elbow is pointing to the ceiling and your hand brushes against your waist. Lower the weight slowly back down.

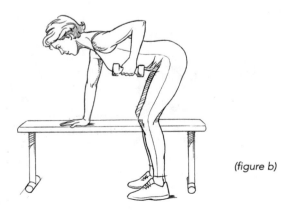

(figure b)

Pullover

(figure a)

Holding a single dumbbell with both hands, lie on a bench, an aerobic step, or the floor with your feet flat and your arms directly over your shoulders. Turn your palms up so that one end of the dumbbell is resting on the gap between your palms and the other end is hanging down over your face. Pull in your abdominals but make sure your back is relaxed.

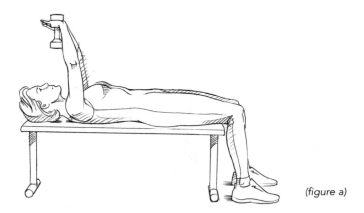

(figure a)

(figure b)

Keeping your elbows slightly bent, lower the weight in an arc-like path behind your head until the bottom end of the dumbbell is directly behind your head. Pull the dumbbell back up overhead, keeping the same slight bend in your elbows through-out the motion.

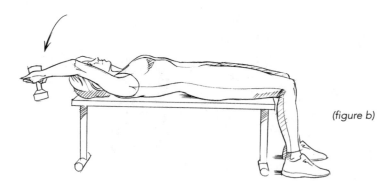

(figure b)

Shoulders

Shoulder Press

(figure a)

Hold a dumbbell in each hand and sit on a bench or chair with back support. Plant your feet firmly on the floor about hip-width apart. Bend your elbows and raise your arms so the dumbbells are at ear level. Pull in your abdominals.

(figure b)

Push the dumbbells up and in until the ends of the dumbbells are nearly touching directly over your head, and then slowly lower the dumbbells back to ear level.

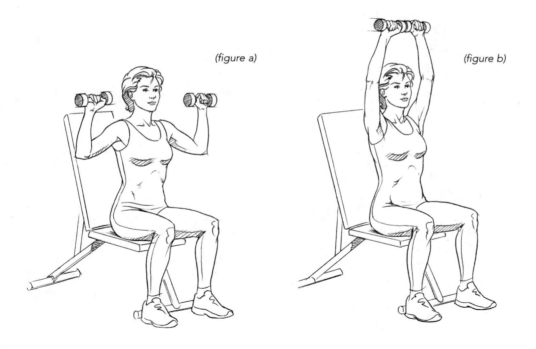

(figure a)   *(figure b)*

Lateral Raise

(figure a)

Hold a dumbbell in each hand and stand up tall with your feet hip-width apart. Bend your elbows a little, turn your palms toward each other, and hold the dumbbells together in front of your thighs. Pull in your abdominals.

(figure b)

Lift your arms up and out to the sides until the dumbbells are just below shoulder height. Slowly lower the weights back down. It may help to imagine that you're "airing out" your armpits as you raise the weight.

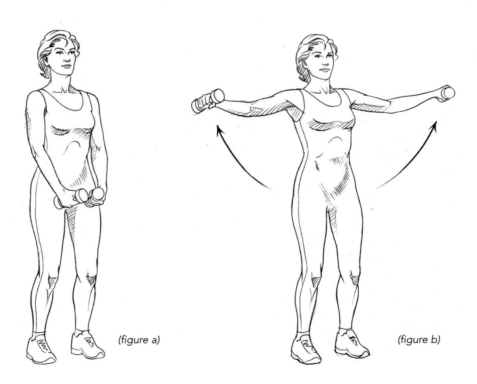

(figure a)   *(figure b)*

Biceps (Front of Arms)

Dumbbell Biceps Curls
(figure a)
Hold a dumbbell in each hand and stand tall with your feet hip-width apart. Let your arms hang down at your sides with your palms facing in.

(figure b)
Curl your left arm up twisting your palm as you go so that it faces the front of your shoulder at the top of the movement. Slowly lower the dumbbell back down, and then repeat with your right arm. Continue alternating until you've completed the set.

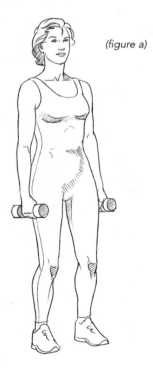
(figure a)

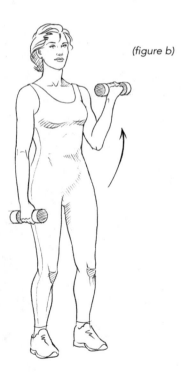
(figure b)

Concentration Curls

(figure a)

Hold a dumbbell in your right hand and sit on the edge of a bench or chair with your feet a few inches wider than your hips. Lean forward from your hips and place your right elbow against the inside of your right thigh, just behind your knee. The weight should hang down near the inside of your ankle. Place your left palm on top of your left thigh.

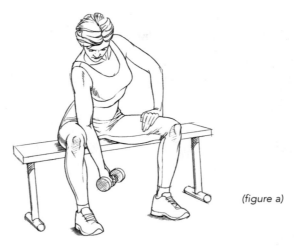

(figure a)

(figure b)

Bend your arm and curl the dumbbell up to your shoulder, and then straighten your arm to lower the weight back down.

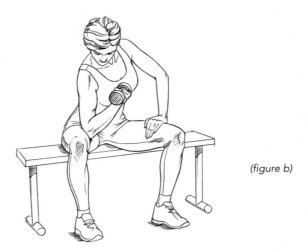

(figure b)

Triceps (Back of Arms)

Kick Backs

(figure a)

Hold a dumbbell in your left hand and stand next to the long side of your bench or chair. Place your right knee on the bench or chair and lean forward at the hips until your upper body is almost parallel to the floor, resting your free hand on top of the bench for support. Turn your left palm in toward your body and bend your elbow up and raise the weight. Pull in your abdominals and relax your knees.

(figure b)

Straighten your arm behind you until the end of the dumbbell is pointing down. Slowly bend your arm to lower the weight. When you've completed the set, switch sides and repeat with your left arm.

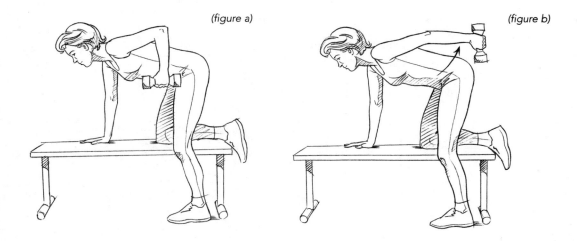

(figure a)   *(figure b)*

Overhead Triceps Press

(figure a)

Sit or stand tall. While holding the dumbbell in one hand raise your arm up overhead. Place your other hand firmly on your elbow for support and to keep your arm stable.

(figure b)

Bend your elbow so that the dumbbell travels diagonally and downward behind your head. Straighten your arm to return to the start. Complete all repetitions and then repeat with the other arm.

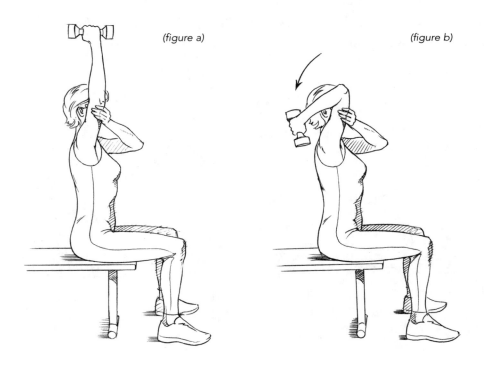

(figure a)   *(figure b)*

Abdominals

Basic Crunch

(figure a)

Lie on the floor with your feet hip-width apart. Cradle your head in your hands without lacing your fingers together and with your elbows rounded slightly inward. Tilt your chin a small way toward your chest and pull in your abdominals.

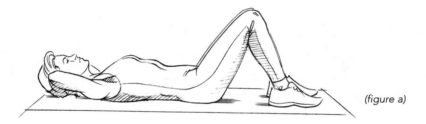

(figure a)

(figure b)

Exhale through your mouth as you curl your head, neck, and shoulders up and forward off the floor. Hold at the top of the movement for a moment, then inhale as you slowly lower down.

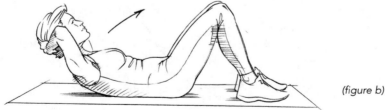

(figure b)

Twist Crunch

(figure a)

Lie on the floor with your feet hip-width apart. Cradle your head in your hands without lacing your fingers together and with your elbows rounded slightly inward. Tilt your chin a small way toward your chest and pull in your abdominals.

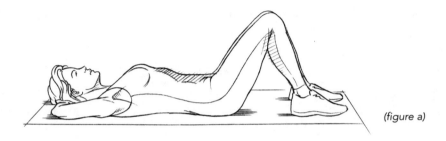

(figure a)

(figure b)

Exhale through your mouth and curl your head, neck, and shoulders up and diagonally toward the right. Hold at the top of the movement, then lower to the start. Twist to the right on the next rep and continue alternating until you complete the set. *Note:* Don't just twist your elbows from side to side. Really concentrate on twisting from your middle as if your waist is a wet towel you are trying to wring dry.

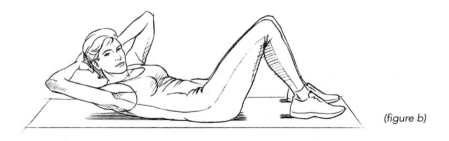

(figure b)

LOSING IT FOR GOOD: WEEK ONE

Starting a new weight loss routine is never easy—especially if you're beginning after a long period of unchecked eating and inactivity. But after the Diet Personality and Fitness Personality assessments, you can feel confident that your individualized diet and workout combination will help you overcome the weight loss issues that hindered you in the past.

Think of this first week as an experiment. Follow your diet and workout routines as directed. Take notes about your progress in your Daily Journals and track your weight and measurements at the end of the week. You may be surprised by your results and how much better you'll start to feel. And that should give you all the motivation you need as you head into Week Two.

Now look up your Week One menu and fitness plans—and let's get started!

Menu Plans

Conquer Your Cravings, page 24

No Time to Diet, page 40

Fitness Plans

Simplicity Rules, page 92

Motivating Moves, page 96

Revved-Up Results, page 100

Don't forget to . . .

- Record what you eat!
- Drink eight eight-ounce glasses of water daily.
- Determine what food items you'll need this week, and stock up.

DAILY JOURNALS: WEEK ONE

Day 1

What I ate today

What I did for exercise

Water count

My moods, challenges, and successes

Today's Pep Talk

It takes time to change years of negative thinking and start feeling good about your body. Here's one way to start: Write down all the activities you engaged in to feel good about your body (walking, taking a bath, giving yourself a manicure). Write down all the positive body behaviors you could engage in tomorrow. Visualize yourself doing these things.

—Ann Kearney-Cooke, Ph.D.

Day 2

What I ate today

What I did for exercise

Water count

My moods, challenges, and successes

Today's Pep Talk

The next time you feel like overeating, try this trick. Look at your watch and try to wait 20 minutes before you eat. In the meantime, take a pen and write down anything that comes to your mind, without editing it. You may gain some insight into why you want to eat more, and after the 20 minutes, you may decide not to overeat.

—Ann Kearney–Cooke, Ph.D.

Day 3

What I ate today

What I did for exercise

Water count

My moods, challenges, and successes

Today's Pep Talk

Try to fit in little things throughout the day. Park your car a little farther away from the building where you work. Walk or at least stand up as much as you can at work. If you can't go outside and walk during your lunch break, find a secluded place inside and do some quick squats, lunges and torso twists. Take a minute or two every hour and give yourself a good stretch, which may not tone your body, but will make you feel better! The little things you do all day really add up.

—L.M., Lose It for Good Community Challenge participant

Day 4

What I ate today

What I did for exercise

Water count

My moods, challenges, and successes

Today's Pep Talk

Don't let others determine what you do for yourself. Be healthy for yourself first, and believe in yourself. We all fail once in awhile, but we get right back up and try again, and you can too!

—J.H., Lose It for Good Community Challenge participant

Day 5

What I ate today

What I did for exercise

Water count

My moods, challenges, and successes

Today's Pep Talk

Once you determine a healthy ideal for yourself, develop a lifestyle to support it. Begin by drawing a circle, and mark the percentage of time you spend each day on daily activities (work, household chores, exercise, relaxation, and so on). Draw a second circle and show how you would need to change your schedule and redistribute your time, to reach your weight loss goals. Maybe it means you have to work less each day or organize a car pool to free up time to exercise. Remember you can't expect different results by continuing to do the same thing.

—Ann Kearney-Cooke, Ph.D.

Day 6

What I ate today

What I did for exercise

Water count

My moods, challenges, and successes

Today's Pep Talk

Determine a realistic weight goal for yourself. Base it on your genetic background, bone structure, age, and so on. Base your weight goal on a healthy ideal versus the beauty ideals of the culture. It's better in the long run to set a lower weight goal that is attainable than a higher one that is unrealistic. Remember, nothing is more motivating than success!

—Ann Kearney-Cooke, Ph.D.

Day 7

What I ate today

What I did for exercise

Water count

My moods, challenges, and successes

Today's Pep Talk

Today is a new day. Define yourself and your body image by what you do each day—not by what was done to you in the past. Let go of negative feelings you have about how you look. It's easier to stay motivated to eat healthy and exercise when you accept yourself.

—Ann Kearney-Cooke, Ph.D.

TAKING MEASURE: WEEK ONE

	Beginning Week One (copy the figures from chart on page 19)	End Week One	Amount of Change
Weight			
Dress size			
Pants size			
Blouse size			
Bust (inches)			
Waist (inches)			
Hips (inches)			
Arms (inches)			
Thighs (inches)			

QUESTIONS AND ANSWERS: WEEK ONE

How Much Cholesterol Is Okay?

Q: I have been looking for information regarding how much cholesterol is safe to consume in one day. My cholesterol is high and I'm not sure what I should be doing besides choosing only no-cholesterol foods and no-fat foods.

—J.B.

A: Current guidelines suggest no more than 200 milligrams of cholesterol each day. That's about the amount in one egg yolk, so it pays to notice from food labels how much cholesterol is in foods. If you keep your meat and chicken intake to no more than four to six ounces per day, and choose very lean cuts, you've got a great start. Avoid fried foods, and keep added fats (such as margarine, sour cream, salad dressings) to a maximum of one teaspoon per meal. Also be careful of crackers, cookies, cakes, and so on—many are loaded with fat.

The amount of fat we eat, especially the amount of saturated fat, is even more important than the amount of cholesterol we consume in terms of keeping our body's blood levels of cholesterol under control.

And there are foods we *should* eat to keep our heart healthy! Fruit and vegetables (five to nine total servings per day), whole grains, and legumes taste great and help lower cholesterol at the same time!

—Lynn Grieger

What About Just Eating Vegetables?

Q: Does broccoli have any fat or calories? Is it possible to diet only on vegetables?

—L.F.

A: We can't live on just one food, or even one type of food, alone. I believe that there are many different types of food on this planet for a reason—we should eat as many of them as possible! Broccoli is a great low-calorie vegetable with no fat, and it's packed with important nutrients, but it's not high in protein. We do need essential fatty acids that you don't find in vegetables; and how long could you really stand to eat only broccoli? Eat many different types of vegetables and fruit, whole grains, and low-fat sources of protein for a balanced diet.

—Lynn Grieger

How Long to Lose This Post-Baby Weight?

Q: I am 35 and just had a baby. I would like to get back to my pre–pregnancy weight. I had a C-section, so I am going to start exercising as soon as my doctor says it's safe. How can I get my stomach back and lose the weight healthfully? My husband says it took 41 weeks to put it on, so I should give myself 41 weeks to get it off. I really need diet help.

—D.S.

A: Your husband is right about the weight not coming off as quickly as you would like. It may even take longer than nine months to lose it, so don't get discouraged. Exercise is a great idea! Combine it with these tips:

- Eat three meals each day. Life can get hectic with a new baby, but take time to eat balanced meals.
- Focus on eating three servings of vegetables and two servings of fruit each day. It's a great start to a balanced meal plan.
- Drink milk or water with meals, and only water between meals. Avoid sweetened beverages such as soda, lemonade, or sugared iced tea.
- Eat snacks only if you are physically hungry. You may be tired, bored, or emotionally drained, but if you're not truly hungry, don't eat.

—Lynn Grieger

Help! I Can't Seem to Get Started!

Q: Help! I need some motivation. I am always saying things like, "I'll start dieting tomorrow." Of course I never do start eating right so I am only left in a constant cycle of overeating. Please help get me motivated by suggesting ways I can improve my unhealthy lifestyle and get out of this slump!

—V.F.

A: Don't get so down on yourself—you can do it! First, take the word "diet" out of your vocabulary. It has become a depressing, intimidating word that implies all or nothing. Start small: Try substituting one unhealthy food with something better for you, and go from there. It'll take a little planning to keep healthy stuff available, but it's worth it. Think of it as a positive shift of your lifestyle, instead of a "diet." And whatever the result, please do not allow how you look to alter how you feel about yourself! Your true assets (personality, sense of humor, intelligence, compassion) are what matter. Good luck!

—K.E.

What Can I Substitute for Dairy Foods?

Q: I am lactose intolerant. What are some substitutions I can make for the dairy products listed in the No Time to Diet meal plan?

—C.O.

A: You can use lactose-free milk, or try a fortified soy milk substitute. There are also soy cheese and soy yogurt if dairy foods bother you. You could also try taking Lactaid pills with meals that include dairy. These over-the-counter pills contain lactase, the enzyme that breaks down lactose (milk sugars), which most of those who are lactose intolerant are lacking in their systems.

—Lynn Grieger

What Can I Substitute for Certain Foods?

Q: Some of the meal suggestions include items that don't agree with me. Can you suggest alternatives for broccoli, cantaloupe, and bananas?

—B.R.

A: Making substitutions is easy. Instead of broccoli, choose any other dark green vegetable: asparagus, green beans, kale, spinach, or green peppers. Instead of melon, try another orange fruit: peaches, mango, or apricots. Instead of bananas, try any other fruit you desire. One of the keys in long-term weight loss is learning to adapt food plans to fit your likes and needs. As long as you choose replacement foods that are similar in nutrient content, you'll do fine in the long run.

—Lynn Grieger

How Can I Work Out with a Young Child?

Q: My son is now four years old and I still need to lose 40 pounds to get back to my pre-pregnancy weight. My problem is how to ever find the time to work out when taking care of him. Help!

—N.S.

A: It can be difficult to find the time to exercise with a four-year-old running around the house, but let me make a few suggestions. Break up your workouts into smaller mini-sessions throughout the day so you don't have to look for a 30-minute uninterrupted block. Let's face it, how often does that happen in your life?

Try a 10-minute brisk walk in the morning, another in the afternoon, and another in the evening. If you can't get out to do this, march in place or walk up and down a staircase. The point is to keep moving for the entire 10 minutes. Don't worry too much about calorie burn or how hard you're working at first. Just get into the habit of doing it. This increase in activity will really make a difference in your appearance and energy level. Keep it up at least three days a week and I can assure you that you will see some results within six to eight weeks.

—Liz Neporent

What Can I Substitute for Free Weights?

Q: I would like to do some strength training at home, but I can't spend a lot of money buying a set of free weights. Are there any items that I might have at home that would make good substitutes?

—K.H.

A: You can use common household items as an inexpensive alternative to free weights. Take empty soda or cleaning product bottles that fit comfortably in your hand and fill two of them with equal amounts of sand. You don't have to fill the bottles all the way—fill them just enough so that the weight is comfortable, yet slightly challenging. As you gain strength, you can add more sand to the bottles for heavier "weights." One alternative, great for doing bicep curls: Place two to three cans each in two plastic grocery bags. Lift the bags by the handles while doing your curls.

Another very inexpensive choice is exercise bands. You can buy a complete set for less than $10 at sporting goods stores and you can rent or buy a tape or check out a book from your local library to help learn how to use them.

You also can use your body weight for a lot of exercises. Push-ups, crunches, squats, lunges, and dips require no equipment at all and are very effective body shapers.

—Liz Neporent

Why Use a Journal?

Q: Does it really help to keep a journal?

—H.C.

A: An eating and exercise journal absolutely, positively does help when you're stuck in a rut. I use one myself. A journal is effective because it helps you determine your patterns. Once you zero in on some of your bad habits—and perhaps why you have these habits—they are easier to change. I also find that keeping a journal keeps you honest about what you're eating, and sometimes can deter you from eating too much. Who wants to write down that they've eaten an entire bag of cookies? If your fitness and nutrition plans work for you, you now have a written plan for how you've made it happen. If you don't shape up as you would have liked, you also can find the reasons on the pages of your journal.

—Liz Neporent

What About That Hip Flab?

Q: I have pockets of flab around my hips. How can I get rid of them? Or is it even possible?

—B.V.

A: The tendency to store fat on your hips—or any other specific place—is the result of the genes you inherited. The solution is the same no matter where your fat is stored: You've got to reduce your overall body fat levels. Start some regular aerobic exercise (try 30 minutes, three times per week to start) and preferably, do some strength training (twice per week would be good to start) to help increase your metabolism. Working the hip muscles underneath the fat will not magically zap inches from that area, although it *can* help tone that area. Exercise and eat sensibly and nutritiously, and you'll start to look better—and *feel* better as well.

—Liz Neporent

Why Do My Workouts Leave Me Groggy?

Q: The last couple of times that I have worked out, the only thing I could think of doing when I got home was napping. I felt really limp and relaxed and needed to snooze. Is this normal? The aerobic teacher says you should feel refreshed, strong, alive, and ready to take on the world.

—R.B.

A: Ordinarily, you should not feel totally spent after a workout unless you specifically set out to work at a maximum level of intensity. Examine the rest of your life to figure out why you feel so drained after your workouts. Did you get enough sleep last night? Have you eaten anything in the two to three hours before your workout? What else were you doing during the day before your workout?

Have you recently started exercising or recently increased the intensity or frequency of your workouts? All these reasons can cause you to feel exhausted after a workout. Or it could just be that your body is still adapting to your workouts. Eventually, your workouts should pump you full of energy. If they don't after a few months, it's a good idea to check in with your doctor about any medications you may be taking or any other possible medical reasons for your fatigue.

—Liz Neporent

How Can I Eliminate Saddlebags?

Q: I have these little bulges of, well, I don't know if they are fat or muscle or what, but I want them gone. They bulge out just where my hips join my thighs. Any suggestions on how to get rid of them or to tone them up?

—M.Y.

A: Unfortunately for us women, this saddlebag syndrome is a common scenario. This is simply where many women's bodies love to hold fat. You cannot spot reduce this area or selectively zap the fat away by exercising. You can, however, spot tone quite effectively. The muscles you want to target are the abductors (outer thigh muscles) and the gluteus medias and maximus (the side of the hip muscles and buttocks). I recommend three to five workouts a week that last 20–60 minutes each. Do something like walking, jogging, or cycling that uses your legs. The recumbent bike is a good choice because it uses your hip and buttocks muscles more than an upright cycle.

If you have access to a Pilates class, I highly recommend you try it. This yoga-like exercise places a lot of focus on the thighs, buttocks, and abs. It has worked for me and I think it may help you too.

—Liz Neporent

Can I Lose 100 Pounds in a Year?

Q: My sister is getting married next year. I was barely 100 pounds just four years ago, and now I've almost doubled that weight. A lot of family members that

I haven't seen since I put on the weight will be there. Is there any way to lose any weight in this amount of time?

—E.C.

A: If you're asking if you can lose 100 pounds in one year, then the answer is an absolute yes. Start today by searching yourself to answer the question why you gained this much weight so quickly. Are you depressed? Bored? Upset? I strongly urge you to understand this before you go forward. Also check with your doctor to ensure that you don't have a medical condition that is contributing to your weight gain.

Definitely start exercising. Start with 30 minutes of walking every day if you can. It's okay to break it up into a few sessions a day. Do whatever it takes. And increase to up to an hour gradually.

Whatever happens, go to the wedding with your head held high. I'm sure your family loves you whether you're 100 pounds or 200 pounds. You are worth more than a number on a scale.

—Liz Neporent

Note: Remember that you should always ask your doctor before beginning any exercise program, and this is particularly important if you've been sedentary for a while or have gained lots of weight—especially if you're over 40 or have particular health concerns. If your doctor recommends a stress test, schedule it before starting your program.

YOUR DIET COMPANIONS: WEEK ONE

Kim's Diary

Looking back on this wonderful first week, I just have to say *wow!* I tried out the quizzes (I am a *Revved-Up* exerciser with *No Time to Diet,* by the way). I was *so* revved up on the first day that I got up at 5 A.M. and did 45 minutes of low-impact aerobics and weights. It felt great, I felt great, and for a change, I enjoyed myself!

I did well this week with my exercise and I worked out every day. I did a variety of exercises including low impact aerobics, weights, fitness ball, and yoga.

I am feeling very good about myself this time around. I am determined to remain positive, and even if I don't lose a lot of pounds after all is said and done, I will be a stronger, healthier person.

Martha's Diary

As a slow loser with 100 pounds to lose, I may not make a lot of progress in just six weeks. But the program did make me measure my body, which I've been resisting for the past year.

More than anything, this program is serving as one of several means of inspiration in this new lifestyle I am following. After 45 years of trying, I've learned that diets don't work—ideas do! And this program has lots of great ideas.

LOSING IT FOR GOOD: WEEK TWO

What did you learn during your first week? Did certain events motivate you? Did some experiences discourage you? Experts recommend noting these things in a journal, which is why we have provided pages at the beginning of these chapters. Keep track of the small successes and lapses you experience. Soon you'll be able to recognize and avoid those discouraging situations, and seek out the support that keeps you going!

During this second week, focus on making the diet and workout plans work for you. If you need to make substitutions or adjustments, now is the time to try them. The programs are guidelines and can certainly be amended as long as you choose alternate foods with similar nutritional values and activities that work the same muscles and require the same effort. It's also a good time to think about when you do your exercise—are you a morning or evening exerciser? There's no wrong answer, but what feels natural to you is most likely to become part of your regular routine.

Now look up your Week Two menu and fitness plans.

Menu Plans	Fitness Plans
Conquer Your Cravings, page 31	*Simplicity Rules,* page 93
No Time to Diet, page 47	*Motivating Moves,* page 97
	Revved-Up Results, page 101

Don't Forget to . . .
- Record what you eat!
- Drink eight eight-ounce glasses of water daily.
- Determine what food items you'll need this week, and stock up.

DAILY JOURNALS: WEEK TWO

Day 1

What I ate today

What I did for exercise

Water count

My moods, challenges, and successes

Today's Pep Talk

Buy a counter and click it each time you are deliberate about eating when you are hungry, stopping when you are full. Keep track of the clicks each day. Reward yourself with a manicure, new lipstick, or any other calorie-free treat as you increase your clicks each week.

—Ann Kearney-Cooke, Ph.D.

Day 2

What I ate today

What I did for exercise

Water count

My moods, challenges, and successes

Today's Pep Talk

Identify and change habitual negative thoughts about your body. Remember your brain is like a computer. Don't keep programming it in a negative way. When you find yourself thinking in a negative way about yourself, visualize a stop sign and say *stop*. Then replace it with a positive affirmation.

—Ann Kearney-Cooke, Ph.D.

Day 3

What I ate today

What I did for exercise

Water count

My moods, challenges, and successes

Today's Pep Talk

Don't let slow progress slow you down! Just remember that this program is not just about losing weight, although that is a *big* part of it. It's also about being healthy, period. Remind yourself each day, even several times a day, that you are doing something good for yourself.

—A.S., Lose It for Good Community Challenge participant

Day 4

What I ate today

What I did for exercise

Water count

My moods, challenges, and successes

Today's Pep Talk

Sometimes it is helpful to keep a food journal and rate your hunger. Write down what you eat and how hungry you are when you eat it. By doing this, and occasionally looking back at your entries, you'll learn to anticipate when you get hungry and gradually learn to make better food choices. You can also prepare by keeping healthy snacks on hand for when hunger strikes.

—Ann Kearney-Cooke, Ph.D.

Day 5

What I ate today

What I did for exercise

Water count

My moods, challenges, and successes

Today's Pep Talk

Attend an event this weekend where food is being served, for example, a party. Focus on the people, instead of the food. Ask them questions you've always wanted to ask; share something about yourself you've never shared. Fill yourself up with people—maybe you won't need to keep going back to food.

—Ann Kearney-Cooke, Ph.D.

Day 6

What I ate today

What I did for exercise

Water count

My moods, challenges, and successes

Today's Pep Talk

I think it is important to reward ourselves along the way for our achievements. I have been buying myself little things like makeup, workout pants, even a new haircut! When I get this last 10 pounds off I am going all out and buying myself some new clothes and a special sexy outfit.

—H.P., Lose It for Good Community Challenge participant

Day 7

What I ate today

What I did for exercise

Water count

My moods, challenges, and successes

Today's Pep Talk

Surround yourself with people who support the lifestyle changes you are making, and not those who reinforce old, unhealthy habits. It is not your fault if critical people surrounded you early in your life, but it is your responsibility to spend your time with positive people now. Make a list of people you would like to spend more time with. Call one of them today.

—Ann Kearney-Cooke, Ph.D.

TAKING MEASURE: WEEK TWO

	Beginning Week Two (copy the figures from chart on page 133)	End Week Two	Amount of Change
Weight			
Dress size			
Pants size			
Blouse size			
Bust (inches)			
Waist (inches)			
Hips (inches)			
Arms (inches)			
Thighs (inches)			

QUESTIONS AND ANSWERS: WEEK TWO

How Can I Cut Back on Starches?

Q: I hear all this talk about weight loss through cutting back on carbohydrates, and it seems like it really works, but how can you cut back on starches? I'm the type of girl who has a bagel, muffin, or toast for breakfast, sandwich for lunch, and potatoes or pasta with dinner. I love pasta! And I get bored very easily with food. How can I cut back on my carbs, and what can I replace them with?

—K.A.

A: One of the problems with low-carb diets is that you have to give up many of your favorite foods, which is why these plans are hard to stick with over the long haul. And, in fact, there is nothing wrong with eating carbohydrates at each meal—but you'll find that whole-grain carbohydrates will be healthier and more filling, as well. Try 100 percent whole-wheat toast or pasta, for example. And you *can* cut down on portion sizes, and make sure you also eat lean proteins (chicken without skin, lean red meat, fish, legumes, tofu) and lots of veggies at every meal. As a rule of thumb, fill half your plate with nonstarchy veggies, one fourth with starchy, high-carb foods such as bread, pasta, potatoes, or rice, and one fourth with protein.

—Lynn Grieger

Note: If you've been diagnosed as diabetic, your doctor or nutritionist will be able to tell you how many grams of carbohydrates you can eat per day, and in this case it is crucial to limit your carbohydrates to the recommended amounts. If you have any suspicions you are diabetic or if diabetes runs in your family, have your doctor check your blood sugar level.

Which Fats Should I Count?

Q: I have been told conflicting things about following a low-fat lifestyle. Do you watch fat, saturated fat and calories, just the fat, or just saturated fat? How much fat should you have each day?

—K.C.

A: Many health authorities recommend a low-fat diet as a way to prevent heart disease and possibly some types of cancer. Some people find they will lose weight, but only if their total calorie intake decreases. That means watch out for foods that are low in fat, yet high in sugar and calories such as fat-free candy, cookies, ice cream, and so on.

You really only need to pay attention to the total amount of fat you eat. If you cut back on total fat, your intake of saturated fat (typically more solid at room temperature—think chicken fat and butter) will also decrease. Read food labels for the total amount of fat per serving.

The goal typically is to get no more than 30 percent of your total calories from fat, and to try to get some of those in the form of "healthy fats" such as canola or olive oil or the fat found in deep-water fish such as salmon. For most women, that works out to 40 to 50 grams of fat each day. That may seem like a lot, but it can add up quickly. Our plans contain 42 to 50 grams of fat per daily menu.

—Lynn Grieger

Is My Metabolism Slower Because I Used to Be Fat?

Q: Is it true that formerly obese people need fewer calories than people who have never been obese to maintain their weight? I need to lose 10 more pounds but find moderate exercise and cutting calories aren't working.

—C.F.

A: The theory is that some formerly obese people have a slower metabolic rate, meaning that their bodies are more efficient and burn fewer calories. It may be harder for these folks to lose weight because of this effect. Another theory is that when we gain weight, not only do our bodies' fat cells increase in size, but also in number. You can't decrease the number of fat cells you have—only the size of those cells—so some obese people will never be able to get to an "ideal" weight.

What all of this means is that sometimes our "goal weight" is set too low. Look at a healthy weight instead—a weight where you exercise regularly, eat a healthy balanced diet that isn't overly restrictive, feel great, and are happy with yourself. That's your optimum weight.

—Lynn Grieger

Should I Reach for Whole-Wheat or Reduced-Calorie Bread?

Q: I have read that bread made from 100 percent whole wheat is best. However, "light" breads have about half or one-third the calories of a regular slice of whole-wheat bread. Usually the light breads have about the same if not more fiber, but are made from "enriched" wheat flour rather than whole-wheat flour. Is one better than the other?

—C.T.

A: I advocate choosing foods based on their nutrient content and not on their calorie content. Enriched flour is flour that was processed, and during this process some of the nutrients are lost. Enriching the flour supposedly adds back the lost nutrients. Whole grains have not been processed and therefore don't need to be enriched.

Which is better? Hands down, the whole grains. We don't know everything about food, but it does seem that the more natural and less processed the food, the better nutritional value it has. Bottom line? Forget diet or light breads and go for breads that are "whole grain." If you're trying to cut down on bread, make your sandwiches open-face and still enjoy whole grains.

—Lynn Grieger

Note: You'll need to look for the 100 percent whole-wheat label, because breads labeled "wheat" aren't necessarily from whole wheat, even if they are brown in color.

Is Cheese Comparable to Milk?

Q: Does a slice of fat-free cheese have the same nutritional value as a glass of milk?

—G.C.

A: In general, a slice of cheese does not have as much calcium as an eight-ounce glass of milk. Eight ounces of milk has about 300 milligrams of calcium, and one ounce of fat-free cheddar has about 100 milligrams of calcium, compared to one ounce of regular cheddar with 200 milligrams. Of course, the amount may vary a bit from brand to brand; read the label to make sure.

Milk is also fortified with vitamin D, which is necessary to help calcium do its job in our bone structure (although you can also get vitamin D from some daily exposure to sunlight). Cheese is typically made from milk that is not fortified with vitamin D. Don't substitute cheese for milk!

—Lynn Grieger

How Can I Eliminate Tummy Fat?

Q: I have a pouch of fat on my stomach. I am generally pleased with the rest of my body, but this bit is annoying me. I exercise a lot and I do not mind doing a little bit more to get rid of it. Any suggestions for what I should do? I'm open to almost anything.

—L.B.

A: This is actually a pretty common problem for certain body types. You are probably "apple-shaped," meaning you carry your excess weight in your tummy but not on your hips and thighs. Unfortunately there isn't much you can do in the way of spot reducing. You can't do an exercise for your tummy and expect to melt the fat away from that area. Your body doesn't operate that way, I'm sorry to say.

If you are overweight, increasing your aerobic exercise and watching your calories will help reduce your overall weight. And I do recommend doing some abdominal exercises (see page 123), which will tighten up and flatten that area to some extent. These exercises also help improve your posture, which always makes your tummy appear flatter and improves your appearance in general. Try doing abdominal exercises two to four times a week, 8 to 15 reps per set. After a month or so you should see some improvement in the look and tone of your stomach area, even if you don't lose any weight.

—Liz Neporent

Is Exercising Late at Night Bad?

Q: I work long hours and also have a long commute. The only time I can work out during the week is after 9 P.M. I usually exercise for an hour or a little more, shower, relax for 30 minutes or so, and go to bed. I recently read that working out within three hours of going to bed is unhealthy and can disrupt sleep. Occasionally, I do feel a little "wound up" and have trouble falling asleep.

—K.C.

A: If this is the only time you have to work out, then it's better than nothing. In fact, I applaud your dedication. There is certainly nothing unhealthy about working out late at night, although sleeping afterward can be a problem. After your workout, try meditating for 10 to 15 minutes. That should help you relax, slow your metabolism down, and help you get to sleep.

—Liz Neporent

Note: Some studies have suggested that a hot bath 90 minutes before bedtime can help you get to sleep.

I'm Seeing No Results!

Q: I have being trying to lose about 20 pounds for the longest time. I do the Tae Bo workout in the morning for an hour, and weight training at night for about 40 minutes. Some weeks I lose about two pounds but then the following week I gain it back. I feel discouraged most of the time because I don't see results.

—M.F.

A: I know that feeling well! But don't give up, because you're on the right track. Tae Bo is great but I think you would benefit from doing an activity such as running, walking, or cycling. Try substituting one that provides a more intensive cardiovascular workout, and therefore burns more calories.

Also, focus on measurements other than weight. Have you lost inches or body fat percentage? If you don't already, start measuring and tracking these two things.

As you are doing so much to build good, healthy muscle tissue, it is possible that you haven't lost weight because of changes in your body composition. Getting and staying in shape is a lifetime commitment, so don't get discouraged just yet. The changes that take the longest to see usually last the longest.

—Liz Neporent

Could I Be Eating Too Little?

Q: Is it true that if you consume too few calories, your metabolism will be lowered? And if your metabolism is lowered, what kinds of problems might that cause?

—G.R.

A: Your metabolism is in effect your body's furnace. Calories are the fuel that stoke this furnace; the hotter your furnace burns, the more calories it uses up just to keep up with basic functions like digestion, breathing, and so on. Your activity level and the food you eat affect your metabolism. The more activity and exercise you do, the faster your metabolism runs, even when you aren't being active. Activity also builds muscle, and muscle burns more calories than fat. In other words, the more muscle you have, the faster your metabolism. If you don't put enough food in your body, your "furnace" doesn't have anything to keep it going. It goes into a sort of "hibernation" mode by slowing down and using fewer calories. So, yes: If you eat too little, you can slow your metabolism.

—Liz Neporent

Should I Try a Pilates Class?

Q: What about Pilates? They offer it as a class at the gym I have joined, but I don't know too much about it. I build muscle easily, but I don't want to bulk up.

—A.G.

A: Pilates makes you think about the way your body moves and how each segment relates to all of the others. Many people find that it presents less of a physical strain than traditional yoga. As to the question of bulk, it's a common myth that lifting weights will make your muscles swell like balloons. Almost no workout will bulk up most women if done correctly. Pilates, weights, whatever—do what you like and what you enjoy coming back to and I'm sure you'll see great results.

—Liz Neporent

How Long Should I Warm Up and Cool Down?

Q: The treadmill machine I use has warm-up and cool-down features. But lately I have been power walking outside. What is the proper length of time for warm up and cool down?

—F.A.

A: You should do three to five minutes at an easy pace for your warm up and cool down, no matter what type of exercise you're doing. If you're doing a workout that's much longer or harder than usual, you may want to increase that to seven to ten minutes.

—Liz Neporent

YOUR DIET COMPANIONS: WEEK TWO

Kim's Diary

Week Two has gone by and I am still going strong and feeling great. Although I have lost a pound this week and 1½ inches off my hips and 1½ inches off my waist, the best part of this whole thing is the way I feel. The sense of control, strength, and energy I have are wonderful. The pride I feel working toward this healthy goal and the example that I am setting for my kids is very fulfilling.

I have followed the *Conquer Your Cravings* diet this week (with minor adjustments) and have found it to be a satisfying way of eating. I am trying to "honor my hunger" by eating only when I am hungry, eating slowly, and stopping when I am comfortably full. This is huge for me. I have discovered over the last few weeks that I am someone who eats because it's there or because I am stressed instead of because I am hungry. I also eat so fast I miss that full feeling and go straight to stuffed. I am thankful for this chance to learn and discover about myself.

Martha's Diary

The past has proven I am a very slow loser, and so far, my progress has been more on a mental level. I've lost just two pounds over the past two weeks, but I'm not discouraged because this follows a year of stringent discipline (without exercise) during which I lost only 12 pounds. At my current rate, with the help of regular exercise, perhaps I can be 40 to 50 pounds lighter by this time next year.

For those who "don't have time to exercise," please be assured there can be grim results for not making some sort of activity a part of your daily routine. I am fortunate that the only side effects I've experienced are diabetes and a heart scare! But if you start now you may never even face those issues.

LOSING IT FOR GOOD: WEEK THREE

Welcome to your third week! At this point you should have started to see (and feel) some results. Maybe you've lost a few pounds. Perhaps you're less bloated and your clothes are fitting a bit better. You may even have more energy and feel less fatigued doing your daily chores.

That extra energy is one of the nicest side benefits of being in better shape. You're probably noticing that carving out a little time for regular exercise can effectively add a few energized hours to your day. Instead of crashing on the couch at 8 P.M., you may feel alert enough to tackle a project you had been setting aside or to play with the kids. Even better, when you're up and about and not sitting motionless on the couch, you're burning more calories. So the happy, healthy cycle continues!

Of course, it's important to take notes on everything you're learning about your healthy (and unhealthy) habits in your Daily Journal.

Now look up your Week Three menu and fitness plans.

Menu Plans

Conquer Your Cravings, page 24

No Time to Diet, page 40

Fitness Plans

Simplicity Rules, page 92

Motivating Moves, page 96

Revved-Up Results, page 100

Don't forget to . . .

• Record what you eat!

• Drink eight eight-ounce glasses of water daily.

• Determine what food items you'll need this week, and stock up.

DAILY JOURNALS: WEEK THREE

Day 1

What I ate today

What I did for exercise

Water count

My moods, challenges, and successes

Today's Pep Talk

I remember watching an ice skater in the Olympics who fell during her performance. Afterward, the commentator asked her, "What were you thinking as you lay on the ice after your fall?" She said, "My thought was, I have to get up, period." What a great response! Next time you "fall"—for example, overeat—don't beat yourself up. Instead, be like the ice skater and focus on getting back on track.

—Ann Kearney-Cooke, Ph.D.

Day 2

What I ate today

What I did for exercise

Water count

My moods, challenges, and successes

Today's Pep Talk

This is about a lifestyle change, and I'm in it for the long haul. I am "losing it for good" to set a good example for my kids and so I never hold back from fully participating in their lives—even if that means wearing a swimsuit!

—T.L., Lose It for Good Community Challenge participant

Day 3

What I ate today

What I did for exercise

Water count

My moods, challenges, and successes

Today's Pep Talk

Control what you can; forget what you can't. Sometimes because we grew up in a situation where things were out of control or chaotic (for example, with a parent who was alcoholic or depressed), we are determined to control everything in our lives. We set up perfectionist standards for ourselves and others. Learn to let go. Take some pressure off yourself today. If you eat more than you wanted to at one meal, return to normal eating the next meal. Overcoming overeating is not about perfectionism, it's about perseverance.

—Ann Kearney-Cooke, Ph.D.

Day 4

What I ate today

What I did for exercise

Water count

My moods, challenges, and successes

Today's Pep Talk

I am not at my goal yet but well on my way, and I am totally convinced that this time I am going to make it. The best thing of all is that I feel so much better about myself. I am so much more self-assured when I go out now.

—R.W., Lose It for Good Community Challenge participant

Day 5

What I ate today

What I did for exercise

Water count

My moods, challenges, and successes

Today's Pep Talk

Make the time you set aside to exercise a time of renewal and self-care. Invite a friend to walk with you in the park; listen to a motivational tape while you walk on the treadmill. Just being outdoors walking with your child or moving in an aerobic class with other women can be nurturing to you on many levels. Call a friend today and set up an exercise date.

—Ann Kearney-Cooke, Ph.D.

Day 6

What I ate today

What I did for exercise

Water count

My moods, challenges, and successes

Today's Pep Talk

Say "thank you" after a compliment instead of discounting it. Remember, if some-one were to give you a gift, you would look that person in the eye and say "thank you." Be gracious, accept the compliment, and take it. It will not only make you feel better, but the person giving the compliment will feel great too.

—Ann Kearney-Cooke, Ph.D.

Day 7

What I ate today

What I did for exercise

Water count

My moods, challenges, and successes

Today's Pep Talk

Relapses do occur. If you binge at breakfast and tell yourself, "I blew it, I might as well overeat all day and start over tomorrow," you are giving yourself permission to overeat. Instead, say, "I blew it, I am going to brush my teeth and start over at lunch and eat healthy." Recovery from overeating is not about perfection. It's about getting back on track more quickly when you do lapse.

—Ann Kearney-Cooke, Ph.D.

TAKING MEASURE: WEEK THREE

	Beginning Week Three (copy the figures from chart on page 151)	End Week Three	Amount of Change
Weight			
Dress size			
Pants size			
Blouse size			
Bust (inches)			
Waist (inches)			
Hips (inches)			
Arms (inches)			
Thighs (inches)			

QUESTIONS AND ANSWERS: WEEK THREE

What Are the Best Late-Night Snacks?

Q: I know, I know. I shouldn't give into those late-night snack food cravings. But sometimes I do. So, what are the safest food choices for late-night snacking? And what's a reasonable portion?

—C.M.

A: The question really is: Why are you eating? Are you hungry? If you're hungry, is it because you skipped meals, or didn't eat enough dinner? If you're really hungry, I recommend eating foods such as fruit, veggies with low-fat dip, yogurt, popcorn, or even half a sandwich. If you're not hungry, can you satisfy that feeling in another way? Sometimes we eat out of habit, boredom, because others are eating, and so on. Do something else!

As for how much to eat, that's even more difficult. How hungry are you? Eat slowly, savor each bite, and try to take at least 20 minutes for a meal or snack. Then reevaluate your hunger and see if you should eat more. A good goal is 100 to 200 calories for a snack, but only if you're really and truly hungry!

—Lynn Grieger

Should I Really Eat This Much Oatmeal?

Q: Breakfast in several of the plans calls for one cup of oatmeal. Are you serious? That's two servings!

—S.K.

A: Yes, I am serious about a cup of oatmeal! Most people don't eat enough breakfast, which is why they're hungry an hour or two later. Two servings of whole grains for breakfast really sticks to your ribs and gets you going for the day. If you find it's too much, slim down the portions a bit. But if you simply *think* it's too much but your body really likes the additional food, listen to your body!

—Lynn Grieger

Should I Snack Before Breakfast?

Q: The new college semester is starting next week and I will have an 8 A.M. class. I have decided to eat a bigger breakfast (as opposed to a big high-fat dinner), but I can't get to the cafeteria before class. So should I eat some sort of energy bar beforehand even though I'm going to eat breakfast after?

—E.K.

A: Why not just eat breakfast before class? If you can't get to the cafeteria for breakfast (I know, 8 A.M. is early!), try having breakfast in your room. What about a slice of whole-grain toast with peanut butter? Or a bowl of high-fiber cereal and skim milk? If you have a blender you can whip up a smoothie with Carnation Instant Breakfast and fruit, or yogurt and fruit, or even skim milk and fruit. Bars are also an option, as long as you choose wisely. Look for 200 to 300 calories, 10 to 20 grams protein, 30 to 40 grams carbohydrates, and 4 to 8 grams fat for a bar that will give you enough energy to last through the morning.

—Lynn Grieger

How Can I Keep Motivated?

Q: I am 5 foot 9 and weigh 160 pounds. My goal is to lose 20 pounds. Every time I start watching dieting and exercising, I lose my motivation in two weeks because I don't see changes! How can I stay motivated?

—G.T.

A: Here is what works for me: I break my overall weight loss goals into smaller ones. Once I reach my first goal I treat myself to something special. Then I will focus on reaching my next "mini-goal." Setting small, achievable goals makes a big difference!

—K.K., Lose It for Good Community Challenge participant

How Can I Avoid Huge Thigh Muscles?

Q: I play sports regularly. Does running make your thighs bigger? Are there any workouts that can slim down the size of my legs? Any workouts that I should avoid if I am afraid of my thighs getting bigger?

—S.D.

A: If you are predisposed to big leg muscles, any exercise routine will likely build up these muscles. This is a simple fact of genetics. If you're a mesomorph (someone given to a muscular build) then you will see different end results from the person who is an ectomorph (someone with a leaner, less muscular build)— even if you both do the exact same workout. Notice I say "different." Not better or more desirable. We each have our own unique body type and the secret is to look the best you can. However, doing strength training exercises with greater repetitions and lower weights will help you tone without bulking up as much.

—Liz Neporent

Am I Too Heavy to Try Running?

Q: I've lost about 13 pounds, but I'm still nearly 100 pounds overweight. Cardiovascular exercise and weight training have changed my life. Now I want to try running. I am wondering if it will be too much for my joints to bear. I have been doing well in the weight training area and have strong legs. But let's face it, running with this much weight is daunting. Is it safe to try? Any special shoe recommendations?

—G.M.

A: Running when you're overweight is an individual decision. I would say that if you have no joint problems *and* if running doesn't cause joint pain or discomfort, then you can give it a try. I recommend that you do a walk-run combo where you walk for five minutes, run for two, and so on. This will give your body a chance to adjust. If after a few weeks this seems to be working out with no joint pain, you can begin to shorten the walking portion and increase the running portion.

Don't even think about speed for the first month or so—give your body a chance to adjust. As for shoes, get something well cushioned and supportive, specifically made for running. Replace them often—every 250 miles or so. This is more often than I usually recommend but I think heavier runners compress and wear out their shoes faster than lighter runners, and you want to make sure you always have plenty of support.

—Liz Neporent

What Can I Do About Cellulite?

Q: I am young and I know that cellulite can be present on anybody, no matter the age or size. But honestly it is making me very uncomfortable—it is embarrassing to wear a mini-skirt and have cellulite showing. What can be done to minimize cellulite (or preferably, totally abolish it from my thighs)?

—B.C.

A: Cellulite is simply fat that has chosen to store itself in a slightly different pattern than typical fat. Look at your mom, sisters, and other close relatives. Chances are if they are prone to cellulite, it is hereditary to some extent. I'm assuming you're fairly thin. If that's the case, I believe weight lifting will make a big difference for you. You should begin to see differences after about a month to two months of regular workouts. You may never be able to completely banish cellulite but you can certainly reduce it.

—Liz Neporent

What Can I Do to Perk Up My Energy Levels?

Q: Is there anything that I can do about my low levels of energy, such as taking vitamins or eating energy bars? Even when I get enough sleep, I have a hard time exercising because I feel very sluggish. Also, is it okay to exercise with sore muscles?

—T.D.

A: While a nutritional deficiency can make you feel sluggish, taking a multi-vitamin should cover all of your vitamin and mineral requirements. That said, only food can provide energy. That energy comes from calories, something vitamins can't provide (they just help you use the food you eat). Perhaps you are just unmotivated because you don't like the type of exercise you're doing. Are you normally tired or just when it comes to exercising? When you are doing something you consider fun, can you keep going for long periods of time without stopping? I'm not just talking about exercise; I mean any activity.

If you think you are bored with the type of exercise routine you've chosen, then try something that's exercise but doesn't seem like exercise, like inline skating, or taking a walk in a pretty place like the beach or woods.

As for soreness, if you work out when you're a little sore, you're probably okay. But if you can't walk properly or lift a pencil without wincing in agony, then you overdid your workout and should lay off until the pain subsides. And if your tiredness continues without apparent cause, check with your doctor.

—Liz Neporent

How Can I Stay Fit While Injured?

Q: I'm so bummed! I have not worked out for a little over a week now because of a recurring neck/shoulder injury. I fell down the stairs at work and so I had to start going back to the chiropractor. What can I do in the meantime to maintain my fitness levels?

—S.E.

A: I took a little fall too. I was jogging along to an appointment with my hands in my pockets when I tripped over nothing (absolutely nothing) and fell flat on my face. I reopened a fracture to my nose from a previous injury, sprained my wrist, bruised my knees to the bone, gave myself a monstrous black eye, and had a face full of abrasions. For about 10 days, I looked as if tigers had mauled me.

The worst part was that I was unable to run or do my other normal activities for about a week. I was going to feel sorry for myself when I realized I had probably been handed an opportunity to rest my body and to work on some aspects of fitness I tend to ignore, such as stretching. By the time I got back on the road, instead of feeling lousy, I felt great. I kept it all in perspective and definitely kept my one good eye on the big picture. This might be a good attitude to cultivate to get you through this down period. A little stretching or yoga might be just what the doctor ordered.

—Liz Neporent

How Do I Start Strength Training?

Q: I am 37 years old, 5 foot 3, 195 pounds, and I had a C-section four years ago. I have no idea where to begin with strength training. Do I do low weight and lots of reps, or high weight and low reps to get the best results? I have what you call an apple-shaped body.

—F.M.

A: Because you are apple shaped, you may be at higher risk for metabolic problems such as diabetes. Since this is the case and because you want to shape up, I recommend getting in plenty of regular cardiovascular exercise such as walking, jogging, cycling, or any other sustained activity. Cardiovascular workouts will not only protect your heart, they will help you maintain a healthy weight. The good news is that most apple shapes tend to lose weight through the middle where extra weight tends to settle. You're more likely to "lose it where you need it" than someone of a different body type.

Weight training is also an excellent thing to do for your health and appearance. I recommend using moderate weight for 12 to 15 reps, two to three sets per body area to start.

—Liz Neporent

YOUR DIET COMPANIONS: WEEK THREE

Kim's Diary

Week Three is done and I am still really gung-ho. I turned 31 this week and I received new workout tapes, a weight bench, and a gift certificate for a full body massage. I am thrilled with the gifts—and with the support my friends and family are all giving me.

I've managed to add more cardio into my workouts this week, and I have created a mini-goal: I want to increase my endurance. I could easily lift weights and do yoga all day, but any kind of full-on cardio is very difficult for me. I get winded and exhausted! So I hope to work on that and see some improvement during the next three weeks of the challenge.

The more I exercise, the more aware I am of what I put in my mouth. I am working on the "no-guilt" theory and running with it. The theory is that if you don't beat yourself up over every little unhealthy thing that you eat (my birthday cake being a great example), you will actually eat less junk since guilt often leads to binges and that *oh-well-I-have-already-blown-it-why-not-one-more* syndrome.

Martha's Diary

On Saturday night, my husband and I went out to dinner—his idea. I was really reluctant; he almost had to drag me. (That is new!) He wanted Mexican food and that's usually hard for me. I find it's really hard to make good choices in a Mexican restaurant because no matter how you cut it, it's about a day's calories if you get a normal meal.

Something must have happened to my brain. I was searching the menu for a new slant on what to order. I ended up with veggie quesadillas, which are stuffed with spinach and cheese, but not a lot. I only ate two-thirds of the rest before I was almost intolerably stuffed!

Driving home with the take-home box, I started thinking about the boxes already in the fridge (from previous nights). I came to the conclusion that I can no longer have my leftovers wrapped up to go because I just end up throwing the food away. Not too long ago, I would have used these take-home boxes for midnight snacks. Now I need to spend afternoons cleaning out the fridge and getting rid of all that food. That's progress!

LOSING IT FOR GOOD: WEEK FOUR

Congratulations, you've passed the halfway point! It's time to give yourself a much-deserved treat. Bubble bath? Book? Beauty treatment? The reward you choose is up to you—but make it a good (and healthy) one!

Now that you're starting your fourth week, you may notice that you're hitting a plateau. If you are frustrated because you see that the pounds have stopped coming off and the tape measure won't budge, you may want to try a week on *Jump Start Your Diet,* which you'll find on page 55. Lynn Grieger created this reduced-calorie plan to give your metabolism a little kick whenever you feel you've stopped making progress. One week should do the trick—then simply return to your regular plan, recharged and ready to lose!

Now look up your Week Four menu and fitness plans.

Menu Plans

Conquer Your Cravings, page 31

No Time to Diet, page 47

Fitness Plans

Simplicity Rules, page 93

Motivating Moves, page 97

Revved-Up Results, page 101

Don't forget to . . .

- Record what you eat!
- Drink eight eight-ounce glasses of water daily.
- Determine what food items you'll need this week, and stock up.

DAILY JOURNALS: WEEK FOUR

Day 1

What I ate today

What I did for exercise

Water count

My moods, challenges, and successes

Today's Pep Talk

When you find yourself knowing the healthy food choices to make but not being able to make them, try this surprisingly powerful trick: Visualize a stop sign and tell yourself to stop. Try to figure out if you're confusing a need for sleep or something to drink with cravings for unhealthy food.

—Ann Kearney-Cooke, Ph.D.

Day 2

What I ate today

What I did for exercise

Water count

My moods, challenges, and successes

Today's Pep Talk

Find role models of women who feel good about their bodies. I went to see Tina Turner in concert this past summer. Although she was dancing next to women half her age, all eyes were glued on her. Why? She had some attitude. She wasn't apologizing for her age or her body; she was strutting her stuff across the stage. Her energy was inspiring. Next time you are feeling self-conscious about your body, think of Tina Turner. Show some attitude—and move through the world with confidence.

—Ann Kearney-Cooke, Ph.D.

Day 3

What I ate today

What I did for exercise

Water count

My moods, challenges, and successes

Today's Pep Talk

When the scale hasn't moved, it doesn't mean you haven't lost anything. People tend to forget that muscle weighs more than fat. So if you have stayed the same weight but lost inches, that's even better than losing pounds. Watching your inches is key to success. If I see inches go, it inspires me to keep doing what I am doing.

—L.G., Lose It for Good Community Challenge participant

Day 4

What I ate today

What I did for exercise

Water count

My moods, challenges, and successes

Today's Pep Talk

We all wish others could just read our minds and know how to support us. But the reality is we have to teach others how to support us in our efforts to change. Tell your partner, "You can help me by watching the kids while I run three times a week." Talk to your friend about meeting to walk on Saturday instead of going out to lunch. Who do you need to talk to about ways to support you in your weight loss goals? Call one of them today.

—Ann Kearney-Cooke, Ph.D.

Day 5

What I ate today

What I did for exercise

Water count

My moods, challenges, and successes

Today's Pep Talk

If we let our slip-ups consume us, then we can never succeed. I just brush myself off, realize it doesn't mean that I've ruined everything, and get back on the old wagon!

—K.B., Lose It for Good Community Challenge participant

Day 6

What I ate today

What I did for exercise

Water count

My moods, challenges, and successes

Today's Pep Talk

Changing the way you eat and exercise is a difficult challenge. There may be days you want to throw in the towel and give up. It's often during these times that you are about to make a major shift in your behavior. Keep in mind the comedic response to "How do you get to Carnegie Hall?" The answer: "Practice, practice, practice." Don't give up. Keep practicing and you will reach your goal.

—Ann Kearney-Cooke, Ph.D.

Day 7

What I ate today

What I did for exercise

Water count

My moods, challenges, and successes

Today's Pep Talk

If you're stuck on a plateau, remember that you must want to make some kind of changes in your life or you wouldn't be here. You just have to look deep inside and ask yourself what is holding you back from achieving your goals. You deserve to be happy and you can be.

—H.P., Lose It for Good Community Challenge participant

TAKING MEASURE: WEEK FOUR

	Beginning Week Four (copy the figures from chart on page 169)	End Week Four	Amount of Change
Weight			
Dress size			
Pants size			
Blouse size			
Bust (inches)			
Waist (inches)			
Hips (inches)			
Arms (inches)			
Thighs (inches)			

QUESTIONS AND ANSWERS: WEEK FOUR

I'm Dreaming of Cheeseburgers and Ribs!

Q: I have horrible protein cravings. All I can think about are cheeseburgers, barbecued ribs, tacos, sloppy Joes, grilled steak, and the like. I eat a variety of foods every day, trying to have a little bit of everything, but if my dinner plans are for fish or pasta, I usually ditch those plans and grill up some burgers, or go to Burger King, or get a sack of tacos. I love fish and chicken, but my body seems to want red meat even more. What can I do to squelch these cravings?

—T.S.

A: Is there anything else different in your life? Try keeping a food diary, and write down everything you eat and drink plus how you feel about these choices. Perhaps you're not eating enough during the day, or maybe you're going through a particularly stressful time—there could be a variety of reasons.

If you can eat these meats in moderate portions, you'll be better off in the long run. Eat slowly, don't feel bad about your food choices, and remember it's the overall quality of your diet that really counts.

—Lynn Grieger

Note: When you "give in" to your red meat cravings, choose healthier options such as steak or other grilled beef—try to minimize the fattier choices such as cheeseburgers.

When Do I Start Seeing Results?

Q: I've been religious about the diet and exercise plan for a couple of weeks, but I haven't seen any results. Is that normal? How long should I allow?

—K.E.

A: The best I can say is to give it a chance. Every body reacts differently to changes in food intake and exercise, and it may take yours a bit longer. Or perhaps you've not seen a change on the scale, but there might be other changes happening—increase in energy level, increase in healthy food intake, decrease in junk food, and so on, that have benefits that may not show up on the scale or tape measure. I would give the program the entire six weeks before you make a decision about continuing.

—Lynn Grieger

Eat Before Aerobics or After?

Q: I am taking an aerobics class twice a week and it starts at 8 A.M. I usually wake up around 7:15 A.M., then head to class at around 7:30. So I have no time for breakfast. Is it better to eat before my aerobics class or after? Will I burn more calories if I eat after or not?

—S.O.

A: Whether you eat before or after exercising won't affect the number of calories you burn, but having breakfast first might give you more energy and endurance. Some people prefer to just drink a glass of juice or perhaps have a piece of toast or yogurt—something quick and easy to digest. If you choose toast, avoid high-fat toppings such as butter or cream cheese (use a little jam or jelly, or a thin spread of peanut butter). If you eat this 30 to 45 minutes before your class starts, you should be fine. Be sure to drink water during exercise: about a half cup (four ounces) every 15 minutes.

When you're done exercising, drink another eight ounces or so of water. If you find that you are absolutely starving after exercising, it will be easy to overeat. Try to eat something light, but that will carry you through the next few hours. Hot oatmeal (avoid the sugared flavored types), fruit, milk, and whole-grain cold cereal are all good choices.

—Lynn Grieger

Am I Eating Dinner Too Late?

Q: How late is too late to eat dinner? Does it really affect your weight the later you eat?

—T.J.

A: I don't believe that there is one cut-off time for dinner. Most of the time when you hear things like "no eating after 7 P.M.," it's designed to cut down on late-night snacking. Eating dinner late does pose problems: If there's a lot of time between lunch and dinner we might find ourselves snacking too much or tending to overeat at supper.

I encourage people to eat the majority of their calories when they are the most active. If you're very active in the evening, then eating a late, larger dinner might make sense. For me, I'm busiest and most physically active in the morning and afternoon. Breakfast and lunch are my big meals, and I tend to eat a lighter dinner. Instead of getting hung up on the time you eat, look at the rest of your day and your meals.

—Lynn Grieger

Do I Need Lower-Body Weight Training?

Q: My primary means of exercise is step aerobics, which I do two to three days per week for 45 minutes. I also routinely take the stairs instead of the elevator at work (about 25 flights per day). In addition to walking for 60 minutes at least two days per week, I do some upper-body weight training (arms, shoulders, back, abs) two to three days per week. Should I add lower-body weight training to my routine, or is all the stepping sufficient?

—R.O.

A: Is it absolutely crucial to add lower-body weight training to your routine? No. Would it make you stronger and probably help protect you from knee injuries? More than likely, yes. Adding in two sets of squats or lunges every time you do your weights would probably be sufficient.

—Liz Neporent

My Job Requires Sitting All Day

Q: I am watching what I eat, changing my eating habits, and walking with weights on a daily basis, but I sit at a desk all day long. I rarely have a chance to get up—I'm supposed to stay in my area all day. I am sitting on my rear end for seven hours a day. Is there anything I can do to firm while I am sitting here?

—C.B.

A: You have hit upon one of the biggest dilemmas of the modern world. Your job requires sitting for long periods of time, but it's hard to stay fit if you don't get to move a lot. I'm not sure if you can do this in your situation, but I highly recommend getting up once per hour (at least) to walk around, clear your head, stretch your legs and get your blood flowing again. You will be more productive because you'll feel better.

While in your chair, you can do some stretches, butt squeezes, and isometric ab exercises that can actually be quite effective. You can also stand for a while. If it's not too intrusive, you can do standing leg raises to the side or back—this is a good trick to use while you're on the phone. Because you sit so much it's even more essential to get in your regular workouts of cardio and weight training. They're going to be the key to keeping your weight down and your muscles from turning to jelly.

—Liz Neporent

What Routines Work Best for Big Bellies?

Q: I would really like to know what cardio routines are best for big bellies. I am 5 foot 4 and weigh 195 pounds. Almost all of that weight is in my upper middle section and I don't know how to get rid of it. I am only walking right now, and something tells me that isn't going to cut it.

—S.C.

A: You're wrong about one thing—walking *can* help you lose weight. Several studies have shown that many people who have lost weight successfully and kept it off have used walking as their primary activity. But (there's always a *but,* isn't there?) you have to do a lot of walking and you have to be consistent. Your aim should be to burn about 2,000 calories a week with any type of exercise.

Walking is such a great exercise because you can do it for a long time without stopping and you rarely get injured. For someone your weight, it would take about 5½ hours of walking a week to burn 2,000 calories. (You burn six to seven calories a minute.) I know that sounds like a lot, but it's a small price to pay—and of course you don't do it all at one time!

—Liz Neporent

Should I Be Sore After Weight Training?

Q: When I first started strength training at my gym, I felt sore for a couple of days following my workouts. Now, a few weeks later, I don't feel sore the next day but I do work my muscles to fatigue. Do you need to feel sore the next day to get the benefit of weight training?

—T.E.

A: Soreness comes from throwing something at your body that it isn't used to. So even if you're in great shape and you try something new, you're going to feel soreness. Once your body becomes familiar with the activity it has the defenses to prevent soreness. This is a good thing. Otherwise you'd be sore all the time.

So even though you're no longer feeling sore after your workouts, you're still getting a good workout. If you feel like you're working hard during your lifting session and pushing yourself to the point of fatigue, you're getting all of the benefits, and probably all of the results, you're after. Whenever you change your routine, there is a decent chance you'll experience a bit of residual soreness.

—Liz Neporent

How Long between Sets?

Q: When I'm doing strength training at the gym, should the time between sets be 30 seconds or 60 seconds?

—R.T.

A: Rest longer in between sets if your goal is maximum strength and a slightly larger muscle. Rest less time if your goal is more tone and calorie burning. You might even cut out your rest altogether if you want to make your weight training a sort of hybrid activity between aerobics and resistance training.

—Liz Neporent

YOUR DIET COMPANIONS: WEEK FOUR

Kim's Diary

This past week has certainly confirmed that I am a stress eater—no question about that! I have decided to create daily "mini-goals" for the next few weeks to see if I can get back up to speed and to push myself a bit. These small challenges include increasing my water intake, boosting my self-esteem, pampering myself, and fitting in extra exercise.

Martha's Diary

Just when you think things can't get any better, they do! I had an "exercise break-through" this week. I've really been pushing myself to do my daily workouts, but I've never enjoyed them. I felt like a gerbil in a wheel. I'd find myself wishing the session was over within the first couple of minutes. My body would also protest with aches and stiffness. Then on Tuesday, I decided to up the pace and take my hands off the rails, thinking I'd last maybe two minutes. But for once this exercise seemed to have a purpose. But I needed something to do with my hands, so I got the weights out. I kept trying to stop myself short of the 20 minutes (in five-minute increments), but once I'd reach the next increment I'd commit to the next until the 20 minutes was up. It was wonderful!

LOSING IT FOR GOOD: WEEK FIVE

At this point you should have started to notice another side benefit of regular exercise and good nutrition—you're probably in a better mood.

Exercise causes the brain to produce chemicals called endorphins that make you feel great (in fact, falling in love triggers the same kind of response). This is what some people refer to as a "runner's high." In addition, eating healthy, balanced meals at regular intervals helps regulate your blood sugar levels, eliminating the spikes and dips that can bring on nasty mood swings. To top it all off, you're probably seeing positive changes in your body and feeling more confident because of it.

Definitely write about your favorite feel-good moments in your journal. And don't spare the details. By reviewing your entries, you may see a pattern and get hooked on your healthy new ways for life!

Now look up your Week Five menu and fitness plans.

Menu Plans	Fitness Plans
Conquer Your Cravings, page 24	*Simplicity Rules,* page 92
No Time to Diet, page 40	*Motivating Moves,* page 96
	Revved-Up Results, page 100

Don't forget to . . .
- Record what you eat!
- Drink eight eight-ounce glasses of water daily.
- Determine what food items you'll need this week, and stock up.

DAILY JOURNALS: WEEK FIVE

Day 1

What I ate today

What I did for exercise

Water count

My moods, challenges, and successes

Today's Pep Talk

Eat in a mindful way today. Each time you sit down to eat, put a spotlight on your eating. Light a candle, turn on the answering machine, and focus on the meal. Be aware of how the food smells, tastes, and sounds as you eat it. Enjoy the food. Focus on mindful eating at one meal each day.

—Ann Kearney-Cooke, Ph.D.

Day 2

What I ate today

What I did for exercise

Water count

My moods, challenges, and successes

Today's Pep Talk

Are you craving sweets? Finding it hard not to stop in the bakery on the way to work? Think of this: "Desserts" spelled backwards is "stressed." Are you working too many hours? Do you have too many responsibilities? Do you feel stressed and exhausted most of the time? Make a list of the demands in your life and the resources you have to deal with those demands. You may have to decrease your demands or increase your resources because you may be turning to high-calorie desserts to numb yourself from the stressful lifestyle you are living.

—Ann Kearney-Cooke, Ph.D.

Day 3

What I ate today

What I did for exercise

Water count

My moods, challenges, and successes

Today's Pep Talk

We all want to have a "perfect body," but that should mean both inside and out. And maybe, just maybe, once we get our insides strong and healthy and craving movement, good nourishment, hydration, and rest, our outsides will begin to change for the better as well. It did not take us six weeks to get the way we are, and it will take longer than six weeks to reclaim our bodies. Keep the faith and keep on keeping on!

—K.D., Lose It for Good Community Challenge participant

Day 4

What I ate today

What I did for exercise

Water count

My moods, challenges, and successes

Today's Pep Talk

If I'm stressed or unhappy, the first thing I'm tempted to do is eat. There are a couple of things I do to fight that urge. First, if I have time, I go for a walk. If I don't have time to walk, I have a cup of tea (coffee would work, too). There's something about drinking a hot drink that seems to fill me up so that I'm not so hungry anymore. If I am at the lowest of the low points and completely out of my mind and I *have* to eat something, I force myself to drink a 16-ounce glass of water before I take the first bite.

—M.G., Lose It for Good Community Challenge participant

Day 5

What I ate today

What I did for exercise

Water count

My moods, challenges, and successes

Today's Pep Talk

We tend to think of all the energy required to make a change in our lives and forget how much suffering accompanies the pain of being stuck. It takes a surprising amount of energy to avoid an issue or to procrastinate on a decision. Is hanging on to self-destructive habits really easier? Would it take the same amount of energy to take the first step in the change process? Would it ultimately free up energy for success?

—Ann Kearney-Cooke, Ph.D.

Day 6

What I ate today

What I did for exercise

Water count

My moods, challenges, and successes

Today's Pep Talk

Teach others how to talk about and treat your body. Remember, your brain is like a computer. When someone makes a negative comment about your appearance, instead of being embarrassed and trying to explain yourself, switch the burden of explanation to the person making the comment. For example, if a person says, "It looks like you've gained weight," in reply ask, "So why are you are telling me I gained weight?" That sort of response will decrease the number of critical remarks others make about your body, and lessen the effect on you.

—Ann Kearney-Cooke, Ph.D.

Day 7

What I ate today

What I did for exercise

Water count

My moods, challenges, and successes

Today's Pep Talk

A lobster periodically outgrows its shell and must move out and exist unprotected in the sea for 72 hours, vulnerable to coral reefs and predators, until its new shell forms. If the lobster doesn't take this drastic, risky step, it will die, suffocated by its confining shell. Have you outgrown your shell? Do you need to be courageous and try something different? Try kickboxing. Train for a three-day hike. Sometimes we are unmotivated because we've outgrown our shell and don't have the courage to shed it and try something new. Be adventurous; try something new today.

—Ann Kearney-Cooke, Ph.D.

TAKING MEASURE: WEEK FIVE

	Beginning Week Five (copy the figures from chart on page 187)	End Week Five	Amount of Change
Weight			
Dress size			
Pants size			
Blouse size			
Bust (inches)			
Waist (inches)			
Hips (inches)			
Arms (inches)			
Thighs (inches)			

QUESTIONS AND ANSWERS: WEEK FIVE

How Can I Cut Back on Sugar?

Q: I have always eaten unhealthy amounts of sugary foods: cookies, candy, soda, you name it. I have to have sweets every day or I feel deprived. All I can think of is something sweet and how to get it. I want to make a serious effort to cut down on the amount of sugar in my diet but I need some advice.

—B.C.

A: We are born liking sugar and sweet foods. How often we eat these types of foods when young also helps determine our eating habits as adults. You can either go cold turkey, or try to cut back on the amount of sweet foods you eat. I would avoid sugar substitutes, since they just maintain our need for sweets. Instead of denying yourself sweets, choose smaller portions, eat them slowly and savor the flavor, and make sure you truly experience the entire sensory event that surrounds eating these treats.

There often is also an emotional aspect attached to our desire for sweet foods. Sometimes we associate good memories with eating sweets, or we've learned to console ourselves with a cookie or ice cream. Try to figure out why you're eating these foods, and be as specific as possible. Then you can take steps to change this behavior.

—Lynn Grieger

Do I Eat Too Much Cereal?

Q: I love cereal! I eat it for breakfast and also to snack on throughout the day. I look for cereals low in sugar and high in fiber. I was wondering if this is considered a healthy habit and if so, what should I look for when purchasing a cereal?

—J.B.

A: You're off to a good start if you choose higher fiber (more than 5 grams fiber per serving) and lower sugar (less than 8 grams sugar per serving) cereals. Add skim milk and you've got a healthy meal or snack! Be sure, though, that you're checking the serving size of your cereal—even healthy foods can pack plenty of calories if eaten in too large portions.

Here's something else to consider: Studies have shown that people who routinely eat fortified breakfast cereal have higher intakes of many vitamins and minerals. If you choose highly fortified cereals and eat more than one serving per day, you could be getting too much of some vitamins and minerals.

If you eat cereal more than once each day, look for cereals with less fortification. Read the labels—if the cereal provides 100 percent of most vitamins and minerals per serving, limit yourself to one serving per day; if it provides 50 percent of most vitamins and minerals, limit yourself to two servings per day, and so on. If you regularly eat these fortified cereals, you may not need any additional multivitamin/mineral supplements. Make sure that you are also eating plenty of fruits, vegetables, and protein foods for a balanced diet.

—Lynn Grieger

How Can I Eat Well on the Road?

Q: Is there such a thing as healthy eating while on the road? I spend 90 percent of my job driving in a car or in airports. I've found a few things that are quick and healthy, but there doesn't seem to be much selection. Any suggestions?

—S.S.

A: It's definitely not easy! However, there are a few things you can do. Try to stop at large grocery stores, which almost always have a deli section or even a salad or sandwich bar where you can make your lunch or dinner. Travel with a cooler. If you're in your car a lot, look into getting a cooler that plugs into the cigarette lighter so food and drinks stay cold all the time. That way you can bring food for the day, or even a couple of additional meals. Carry fresh fruit in your cooler, too. For flights with meal service, ask in advance for special meals—try vegetarian or heart-healthy, which are almost always tastier and healthier. If the airline offers only snacks, carry your own. Drink plenty of water to avoid loading up on unwanted calories. I have favorite delis in towns I often visit, and I make a point of stopping there even between meals to purchase something for the next meal if I'll be on the road.

—Lynn Grieger

Do I Need to Cut Back on Caffeine?

Q: I enjoy a good cup of coffee some mornings and I drink diet colas regularly. Will all this caffeine intake hinder my weight loss? I do notice that coffee curbs my appetite, but is it a healthy appetite suppressant?

—A.N.

A: Caffeine is the most widely consumed drug in the world. Too much of it can make us tense and anxious, which doesn't help when you're trying to lose weight. Three cups of coffee or two 12-ounce sodas per day are fine for most people. Some people drink coffee or diet soda to feel full without eating extra calories, but this usually backfires with increased hunger later in the day. The solution? Enjoy a cup of coffee in the morning or a diet soda in the afternoon, but make water your beverage of choice.

—Lynn Grieger

Am I Strength Training Too Much?

Q: I currently do strength training exercises 30 minutes a day, seven days a week. I have recently read some articles on strength training that say to do the exercises three days a week. Am I doing it too much? I am trying to stay as toned up as possible.

—M.C.

A: It sounds like you need to take more rest between workouts. It is best to work each muscle group two to three times a week with at least one day of rest in between workouts. Doing more will not help you tone faster and may actually impede your progress. If you are doing the exercises properly and feel tired and challenged by the end of each workout, then your muscles benefit from at least 48 hours of rest, regrowth, and recovery. If you don't give your muscles some rest, you put yourself at risk for injury, strain, and muscle inflammations. You can lift five to six days a week rather than just three. If you decide that you like weight lifting and enjoy an extended schedule, then you should work some muscles on a given day while you rest others. For example, you could work out your upper body and abs on Monday and Wednesday and your lower body on Tuesday and Thursday.

—Liz Neporent

Exactly How Should I Stretch between Sets?

Q: All the articles I've read say you should stretch between sets when doing strength training exercises. They never say what stretches you should do. What stretches should I be doing between sets?

—C.G.

A: The stretches you do between sets should coincide with the muscles you work. For instance, if you've just completed a set of chest exercises, such as push-ups, you want to follow that with a chest stretch—clasping your hands behind your back, lifting your chest up, and pressing your arms up and outward to spread the stretch across your chest and shoulders. After a squat, you want to do a thigh or buttocks stretch. You can do individual stretches between sets if you want, but you can also stretch all your muscle groups after your workout.

—Liz Neporent

What About These Fitness Machines?

Q: Is working out at 80 to 90 rpm on a stationary bike okay for calorie and fat burning? Also, I've recently tried a new machine like an elliptical training machine, but with bars so you can move your arms. I found that I got tired on this one really fast and I was on the lowest level.

—D.T.

A: Any time you burn calories you're burning fat. In fact, here is the absolute rule: The workout that burns the most calories is not only the best fat burner, but it's also the best for weight loss. This is good news. It also means you have choices. If you're in a hurry, you can work out at a high intensity for a shorter period of time. If you don't like the feel of high intensity, you can work out longer at an easier pace.

As for the elliptical trainer with arms, it may burn a few more calories than the one without arms, but probably not many more. You may feel more tired because you're not used to the action or because you haven't previously trained very hard with your upper body. Certainly use it if you enjoy it, but if you prefer other aerobic workouts, do those. Again, for weight loss, it's all about the calories.

—Liz Neporent

Should I Exercise with a Cold?

Q: I've been doing aerobics for one hour per day, three to five days a week, for several weeks. I just caught a cold, and my energy is up and down. Should I lay off exercising until I get over it or should I keep it up? If I lay off, when should I start again?

—L.J.

A: This will sound obvious, but it's so true: If your workout makes you feel worse, then skip it. If it does not make you feel worse or it makes you feel better, then go for it. However, when you're sick, it's not the time to go at it full throttle or try something new and challenging. Get some extra sleep too.

—Liz Neporent

When Will I See Some Benefit to My Abs?

Q: How long does it really take to tone and enhance the abs?

—B.F.

A: Most people will see some changes to their abs after four to six weeks of regular training in the form of some flattening and better muscle tone. If you have no additional fat around your middle, you should see some really significant changes after eight to ten weeks.

However, if you have extra fat around your middle, please understand that all of the ab exercises in the world aren't going to give you that six-pack look. Yes, the exercises will improve your appearance and yes, you will stand up straighter and have better posture because your abs are stronger, but ab exercises do not melt fat away from your middle. The only way to do that is sensible diet and calorie-burning exercise.

—Liz Neporent

How Can I Deal with Allergies?

Q: My allergies have hit hard this season, so hard that I have been laid up for a week. I am trying to train for a five-kilometer race. If I can't get out and run because of allergies running amok, how can I be ready for this race?

—S.E.

A: This is a question for your doctor. Ask if any medications will offer relief while you're wheezing and sneezing during exercise. My other recommendation is to work out on a treadmill in a clean, air-conditioned gym as much as possible. This is usually the best location for allergy sufferers because the air system filters out a lot of the allergens. If that's not an option, plan your exercise for the part of the day when the pollen count is the lowest. Usually the local newspaper or weather channel will describe which parts of the day hold the least trouble for allergy sufferers.

—Liz Neporent

YOUR DIET COMPANIONS: WEEK FIVE

Kim's Diary

I have been doing personal "mini-challenges" each day this week and think it has been a great addition to my day. The toughest one was *Look at yourself, unclothed, and say or think only positive thoughts.* How hard was that? I had to squash the thoughts of "Oh my, that stomach is huge!" and replace them with positive thoughts. My response was, "What a wonderful body I have; it produced my beautiful children." I hope to do this particular exercise each week.

Whenever I got the urge to eat and wasn't sure I was hungry, I sipped a glass of water and waited 20 minutes before reevaluating my hunger. It worked really well. I found that sometimes I was just thirsty—other times I was just bored or stressed.

Martha's Diary

We were in Washington, D.C., almost all week and I learned how difficult it can be to try to maintain a routine while away from home. Breakfasts weren't too difficult because we had complimentary continental breakfasts and I was able to get a bowl of cornflakes each morning, along with a plate of fresh fruit. It went downhill from there, mainly because of what I was doing all day—genealogy research in a library with no place to eat. The first day, I wandered onto the street and got a hot dog and a Diet Pepsi. The second day, it was cheese crackers and a Diet Pepsi. Dinner at night was the really big problem. Every restaurant we tried seemed to have a chef who specialized in making things elegant, expensive, and fattening. I survived the experience by being really careful and consuming only small portions.

On the other hand, exercise went well. I did lots of walking, as the weather was great and I had my tennis shoes along. But it's nice to be back home.

LOSING IT FOR GOOD: WEEK SIX

You're in the home stretch of this six-week program, but are you on your way to reaching your goals? It's time to take stock of all that you've accomplished. Have you made fitness a regular part of your routine? Are you eating more healthfully? Have you lost pounds or inches? Do you have more energy? Has your mood improved? If you've answered yes to these questions, you're on the right track. You can certainly continue using these meal plans and exercise routines in the weeks and months to come—and keep journaling and logging your progress in a notebook of your own.

Once you reach your goals, you can maintain your weight loss by increasing your caloric intake (think eating bigger salads, more vegetables, and a few more healthy snacks, not doubling up on dessert) while keeping up your workout schedule.

Now look up your Week Six menu and fitness plans.

Don't forget to . . .

- Record what you eat!
- Drink eight eight-ounce glasses of water daily.
- Determine what food items you'll need this week, and stock up.

DAILY JOURNALS: WEEK SIX

Day 1

What I ate today

What I did for exercise

Water count

My moods, challenges, and successes

Today's Pep Talk

Fill a cupboard in your house with self-care items. You might put in it the phone numbers of friends to call, inspiring books, great CDs, and messages to fill your soul. The next time you get the urge to dig through the refrigerator, ask yourself if you are really hungry. If you aren't, reach into your "self-care cabinet" and choose one of those calorie-free treats instead.

—Ann Kearney-Cooke, Ph.D.

Day 2

What I ate today

What I did for exercise

Water count

My moods, challenges, and successes

Today's Pep Talk

My mother used to share with me an Irish saying, "It's in the shelter of each other that the people will survive." Take time to develop friendships with people where you celebrate each other's successes and be there for each other during the tough times. When you are excited about a promotion, instead of stopping at the bakery to celebrate, call a friend and celebrate together. When you are feeling bad about yourself, instead of watching television and eating chips, share with someone close to you how you are feeling. Be a "shelter" for each other today.

—Ann Kearney-Cooke, Ph.D.

Day 3

What I ate today

What I did for exercise

Water count

My moods, challenges, and successes

Today's Pep Talk

When you're just starting a program, it can be a little tough. Eating right and exercising feels different at first, sometimes it can even feel kind of bad. But as the weeks pass and you get your routine going, and the compliments start coming in, that's when it starts to feel great. Whenever I have days like that, I write it all down in my journal. What I did, what someone said, what I was wearing. When I'm having a bad day, those entries are the first things I read to get me going again.

—E.L., Lose It for Good Community Challenge participant

Day 4

What I ate today

What I did for exercise

Water count

My moods, challenges, and successes

Today's Pep Talk

Instead of eating grapes for your snack, do you find yourself reaching for the ice cream? Research shows that when people are fatigued or depressed, their ability to make healthy choices decreases. Fatigue can be caused by a lack of sleep, over-stimulation, or simply by having too many things to do. Deprivation can be caused by always giving more than you receive back from others. Make a list of the ways you can decrease the fatigue and deprivation in your life. You might not be making the right choices because you are exhausted—not because you lack discipline.

—Ann Kearney-Cooke, Ph.D.

Day 5

What I ate today

What I did for exercise

Water count

My moods, challenges, and successes

Today's Pep Talk

In any relationship where both individuals are stating what they want, at times what they want will be in conflict. Women often give in and do what others want in order to avoid conflict, which often leads to resentment, anger, and overeating. Learn to negotiate your needs with other people. Try to communicate with others. You may find that over time you are turning to food less often—and turning to people to get your needs met.

—Ann Kearney-Cooke, Ph.D.

Day 6

What I ate today

What I did for exercise

Water count

My moods, challenges, and successes

Today's Pep Talk

Resentment and bitterness get you nowhere. Forgive yourself and others. Remember most people do the best they can with the resources they have. Parents can't teach children what they themselves don't know. Challenge yourself to base your self-esteem on the choices you make each day, not on what was done to you in the past. This applies to eating, too. Don't worry about what you did yesterday—focus on what you're eating today.

—Ann Kearney-Cooke, Ph.D.

Day 7

What I ate today

What I did for exercise

Water count

My moods, challenges, and successes

Today's Pep Talk

Remember a little bit of change each day leads to real change. Take care of the house you live in—your body—by following the tips I shared during this program.

—Ann Kearney-Cooke, Ph.D.

TAKING MEASURE: WEEK SIX

	Beginning Week Six (copy the figures from chart on page 203)	End Week Six	Amount of Change
Weight			
Dress size			
Pants size			
Blouse size			
Bust (inches)			
Waist (inches)			
Hips (inches)			
Arms (inches)			
Thighs (inches)			

QUESTIONS AND ANSWERS: WEEK SIX

Help! I'm Starving in the Late Evening!

Q: I keep pretty long days. I usually get up at 6:40 A.M. for a one-hour workout and then I'm busy all day. The problem is that in the late evening I am starving. Sometimes I can't think about anything else. Usually I snack on crackers, granola bars, or some fruit, but it's not that satisfying. Water and diet sodas don't help either. I'm trying to eat close to 1,500 calories a day but I seem to blow it at night. The other problem is that in the morning when I go to work out, my stomach is growling.

—J.Z.

A: It's often easy to get by on fewer calories during the day when we're busy, but when we get home and are able to relax a bit, suddenly we're starved. Make sure you eat breakfast and lunch. Try to eat balanced meals with some protein, veggies, and complex carbs such as sweet potatoes, brown rice, and whole-wheat pasta, and to eat something before you work out. Try a glass of juice, half an English muffin or bagel with a spread of peanut butter, or half a banana to give you more energy to devote to your workout. Try a low-calorie diet bar (such as the ones Slim-Fast makes) in the evening when you're hungry. Make sure to eat a balanced dinner, as well—add a glass of skim milk and a piece of fruit to the combination I've described for breakfast and lunch. Also, 1,500 calories may be too low for you—and if your 1,500 calories includes all the evening snacks, you'll be better off eating more during the day so you're less likely to snack at night.

—Lynn Grieger

Just Can't Resist French Fries!

Q: I have tried to stop eating French fries, but no matter what, if I run out of time and have to grab a sandwich, I always feel pressured to order them. I know that the fault lies in my lack of planning, but with a full-time job and a full-time school schedule, it's not always easy to pack for two meals a day, especially as I'm not a morning person. I cannot manage to pass up that treat. Please help!

—J.L.

A: Cravings are typically caused by habit, hunger, deprivation, or face-to-face contact. Sometimes even all four are involved. If it's a habit (and it sounds like it is), breaking the habit means starting a new one. Decide you will not order French fries, and instead order a side salad. This will be difficult at first but gets easier with practice. Try to set yourself up so you're not ravenous when you get to the drive-through. Bring a piece of fruit for a snack, eat more breakfast, or try to get to lunch earlier.

Sometimes we feel deprived, and then we go overboard. Maybe you think you really shouldn't eat French fries, but you love them so you eat them. Often writing out your feelings and thoughts in a journal can be helpful.

And sometimes we're simply faced with French fries. You could order a smaller size, share them with a friend, or eat a few and throw out the rest. It's important to remember that ultimately you have a choice here. What do *you* want to do? You can certainly lose weight and still eat French fries, but you'll need to consider how many you're eating and cut back on your food intake somewhere else.

—Lynn Grieger

What's the Scoop on Processed Cheese?

Q: I've heard good and bad (more bad) things about processed foods, but how bad is processed cheese, really? I like Kraft Singles fat-free cheddar cheese slices because they're great for adding melted cheesy flavor, calcium, and protein without all the fat and calories. Should I really consider cutting them off my shopping list?

—S.P.

A: I won't say that all processed foods should be eliminated from our diet, because then we'd really be limiting our food choices. The idea is to choose less-processed foods whenever possible, such as whole-grain bread or brown rice instead of processed white bread or white rice, or baked potatoes instead of a boxed potato mix.

You have some specific reasons why you're using processed fat-free cheese, so it makes sense to go that route. Another choice would be to use regular cheese but less of it. Plus you can choose other less-processed foods, like fruits, vegetables, brown rice, whole-grain bread—and stay away from boxed and canned foods as much as possible. It's all a system of trade-offs and making decisions that are best for you.

—Lynn Grieger

What's Normal Water Retention?

Q: I weighed and measured myself on Monday. I hate to say it but I am exactly an inch larger in my hips, thighs and waist. I am assuming this is due to the fact that it's "that time of the month." How much would be considered water retention? My weight was a pound more than last time but I am thinking the same thing: water.

—S.G.

A: Your weight can fluctuate during your cycle. Some women yo-yo up and down as many as 10 pounds in a month. This can get worse or better as you age depending upon your lifestyle, hormone levels, and so on. The best way to help control this is to drink a lot of water to flush your system, avoid salt (sodium), and eat plenty of fiber. These tactics in combination will help keep bloat to a minimum.

—Liz Neporent

I'm Longing to Wear Tank Tops!

Q: Help! I have flab on my arms. Is there anything that can be done? I am not a large person (I'm 5 foot 3 and weigh 130 pounds) but have always had big arms. I would love to be able to wear tank tops.

—S.A.

A: If your arms are flabby due to excess weight, then doing some extra cardio exercise and watching what you eat can help reduce them. It does not sound like this is the case, though. I think doing some targeted arm exercises such as biceps curls, triceps extensions, and bench dips will greatly improve the tone and appearance of your arms. I recommend two to three workouts a week. After a month you should begin to see a difference.

—Liz Neporent

How Can I Fight a Slump?

Q: I have been doing well with my dieting and exercise. I have 10 or so more pounds to lose, but I'm in a slump. I'm maintaining and gradually losing weight, but I'm getting bored with my exercising. I don't mind working up a sweat, and am currently varying a step routine with some walking and running. Do you have any suggestions?

—D.D.

A: If you're sick of your routine, by all means change it! There are many possibilities. You could join a walking group or find a running buddy, or buy some new videotapes. Try an entirely new activity such as hiking, inline skating, snow shoeing, climbing, or elliptical training. The possibilities are endless. There is no reason to stick with a routine that bores you when there is so much else out there to do!

—Liz Neporent

My Weight Is Creeping Back!

Q: I am close to my goal weight, but the scales have been creeping back up lately. My fitness trainer at the gym says that I'm at a very good state of physical fitness. I do 45 minutes of cardiovascular exercise, three times a week. I take brisk walks frequently (with the dog), and I weight train twice a week. As the mother of a three-year-old and a part-time researcher, I can't do any more than I'm doing.

Is there any way to get the weight back down without negatively affecting my fitness level and lean muscle development?

—G.A.

A: I would start by keeping a food diary to see if anything jumps out at you. You may unknowingly be eating more calories than you realized. It sounds like you're doing a good amount of exercise right now but perhaps you can play with what you're doing within the time frame you have. For instance, if you are riding a bike for your cardiovascular workouts, switch to something different—the treadmill or elliptical trainer. Sometimes you need to make a change to give your body a kick-start in the right direction. Or switch the type of workout. If you typically do the same intensity for the entire 45 minutes, try mixing in some fast intervals of three to five minutes. Or, does your dog feel like jogging a little during his walks?

And try getting some "stealth exercise" in every day by changing a few of your routines. If you normally take an escalator up a few flights of stairs, walk it instead. Stand when you talk on the phone, and whenever possible get up and walk around. I find that some people who are just on the edge of getting where they want can often "tip the scales" in their favor just by adding in a little extra daily movement.

—Liz Neporent

What Can I Do About Cellulite on My Legs?

Q: Is there any way to get rid of cellulite? I am 5 foot 4 and 112 pounds, and I work out three times a week. I am in overall good shape, but I carry fat around my waist from three babies. I have noticed cellulite on the back of my legs for the last several years, even though my legs are toned and muscular. I can live with it, but if there is something I can do without starving myself, I'm willing to try it!

—M.T.

A: Based on your weight, I think you're probably where you need to be in terms of health. Cellulite is simply a fat storage pattern: Fat is hemmed in by collagen fibers, which gives it that "cottage cheese" appearance. It's also one more thing you can blame on your parents, since it's often a matter of genetics. There are many heavy women who don't have any cellulite and plenty of very slim women who do.

In your case, since weight loss is not your problem, toning up a bit more may be the answer. Doing some focused leg-strength training may reduce the appearance of the cellulite. Warning: It will probably take a lot of effort to get rid of it altogether. You seem to have a good, healthy attitude about your body, so don't become obsessed about this.

—Liz Neporent

What About Fat on My Back?

Q: I was trying on clothes a few days ago when I noticed that I have a huge fat roll on either side of my back, about level with my arm pit. How can I get rid of this?

—T.F.

A: This is a common fat storage for women. And if you have extra fat, you've got to burn it off. That means more cardiovascular exercise and less eating. I can't guarantee that you'll lose exclusively from that area, but some of it will come off. In the meantime, some toning exercises can help firm the muscles in that area, which will give it a tighter appearance. A simple exercise such as push-ups targets that area quite nicely. Two to three sets of 8 to 15 reps a couple of times a week will make some differences to your appearance in four to eight weeks. You'll see results more quickly if you work on calorie-burning exercises at the same time.

—Liz Neporent

YOUR DIET COMPANIONS: WEEK SIX

Kim's Diary

Another week has come and gone, and although I wished for a less stressful one, I was granted an even more stressed-out seven days. This time my son became ill and spent three days in the hospital. I did better with my emotional eating despite it all and questioned how hungry I really was before taking a bite. I also managed to squeeze in exercise here and there where I could—I even did yoga in my son's hospital room after he fell asleep.

I didn't eat the healthiest foods (being at the mercy of hospital fare and what others brought to me) but I didn't sit and gorge through my stress either. I actually had the presence of mind to start keeping a water bottle and a handful of teabags in my purse and they came in handy.

I've noticed that I am better at handling that urge to eat when stressed. I'm finding that a nice cup of hot tea works just as well as a candy bar.

Martha's Diary

Here we are at the final week. First of all, 10 pounds have slipped off quietly during the Challenge. I'm exercising on a daily basis and journaling.

My husband's company was having a party over the weekend. I had been dreading the event for weeks, but I finally had to face my insecurities.

The other people in his group are all younger professionals. I've always felt inferior around them because, until recently, I had little interest in maintaining a healthy lifestyle. I'm too old to care about the superficial aspects of thin—I only want good health. I've made progress, but I still wonder if anyone would believe I walk on a treadmill an hour a day.

Well, a buddy told me to march in with an attitude and for once never believe that anyone could look down on me. I did, and had a great evening!

ABOUT THE EDITOR

Emily Lapkin is the director of Diet, Fitness, and Health at iVillage. She lives in New York City.

ABOUT iVILLAGE

Based in New York City, iVillage Inc. was founded in 1995 with the intention of "humanizing cyberspace." In the early years of the Internet, there were few places for women to find solutions and discuss their problems, needs and interests. By providing a clean, well-lit space, iVillage carved out a unique place where women could gather and find information and support on a wide range of topics relevant to their lives.

Today, iVillage is a leading women's media company and the number one source for women's information online. iVillage includes iVillage.com, Women.com, Business Women's Network, Lamaze Publishing, The Newborn Channel, iVillage Solutions, Promotions.com, and Astrology.com.

iVillage.com's content areas include Astrology, Babies, Beauty, Diet & Fitness, Entertainment, Food, Health, Home & Garden, Lamaze, Money, Parenting, Pets, Pregnancy, Relationships, Shopping, and Work.

SHARE YOUR SUCCESS WITH US!

iVillage has always believed that many of the best solutions for problems in women's lives come from other women who've "been there and *solved* that." If you have a success story based on following the Losing It for Good program, we would love to hear about it.

We invite you to become part of our network of advice-giving women and to have your words of wisdom featured in upcoming iVillage Solutions books, by sending your best advice on dieting, weight loss, and fitness to: iVillage Solutions Books, iVillage Inc., 512 Seventh Ave., New York, NY 10018. Or email us at ivillagesolutionsbooks@mail.ivillage.com.

We look forward to hearing your advice, as well as any of your comments and thoughts about our books.